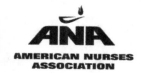

AMERICAN NURSES
ASSOCIATION

M000272214

Scope AND
Standards
OF PRACTICE

Correctional
Nursing

2ND EDITION

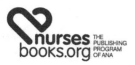

nurses
books.org

THE
PUBLISHING
PROGRAM
OF ANA

American Nurses Association
Silver Spring, MD
2013

American Nurses Association
8515 Georgia Avenue, Suite 400
Silver Spring, MD 20910-3492
1-800-274-4ANA
http://www.NursingWorld.org

Published by Nursesbooks.org
The Publishing Program of ANA
http://www.Nursesbooks.org/

The American Nurses Association (ANA) is a national professional association. This ANA publication—*Correctional Nursing: Scope and Standards of Practice, 2nd Edition*—reflects the thinking of the practice specialty of holistic nursing on various issues and should be reviewed in conjunction with state board of nursing policies and practices. State law, rules, and regulations govern the practice of nursing, while *Correctional Nursing: Scope and Standards of Practice, 2nd Edition*, guides correctional registered nurses in the application of their professional skills and responsibilities.

The American Nurses Association (ANA) is the only full-service professional organization representing the interests of the nation's 3.1 million registered nurses through its constituent/state nurses associations and its organizational affiliates. The ANA advances the nursing profession by fostering high standards of nursing practice, promoting the rights of nurses in the workplace, projecting a positive and realistic view of nursing, and by lobbying the Congress and regulatory agencies on health care issues affecting nurses and the public.

ISBN-13: 978-1-55810-499-0   SAN: 851-3481   06/2014R

Contents

Preface

In 2011 the American Nurses Association (ANA) convened a volunteer work group of correctional nurses tasked with the responsibility of reviewing and revising the 2007 *Corrections Nursing: Scope and Standards of Practice.* The registered nurses and advanced practice registered nurses held various positions in federal, state, and local adult and juvenile correctional and detention facilities as well as academic institutions, professional organizations, and healthcare facilities, and contributed diverse perspectives in all discussions.

The work group used *Code of Ethics for Nurses with Interpretive Statements* (2001); *Nursing's Social Policy Statement: The Essence of the Profession* (2010); and *Nursing: Scope and Standards of Practice,* 2nd Edition (2010) as foundational resources and completed its work via telephone conference calls, and electronic mail communications.

In 2012 a draft document was posted at ANA's web site (www.NursingWorld .org) for a 45-day public comment period. The work group reviewed each resultant comment and further revised the draft as necessary.

In 2013 the ANA Committee on Nursing Practice Standards completed its review of the draft of *Correctional Nursing: Scope and Standards of Practice* against established review criteria. Recommended revisions were completed before the ANA's Board of Directors conducted a final review and approved this nursing specialty scope of practice statement and acknowledged the scope and standards of correctional nursing practice in February 2013.

Contributors

Correctional Nursing Scope and Standards Workgroup

Patricia A. Voermans, MS, RN, APN, CCHP-RN, Chairperson

Patricia A. Blair, PhD, LLM, JD, MSN, CCHP

Jeannie Chesney, MSN, RN, BSN, CCHP-RN

Margaret Collatt, RN, CCHP-A/RN

Collean D'Acquisto, RN, CCNM, CCHP

Laurie Josefek, BSN, RN

JoRene Kerns, BSN, RN, CCHP

Catherine M. Knox, MN, RN, CCHP-RN

Jacqueline Moore, PhD, RN

Mary Muse, MS, RN, CCHP-A, CCHP-RN

Denise M. Panosky, DNP, RN, CNE, CCHP, FCNS

Ellyn Presley, RN, CCHP-RN

Lori E. Roscoe, PhD, MPA, BSN, CCHP-RN

Lorry Schoenly, PhD, RN, CCHP-RN

Bernardine Scott, RN

Nancy Sue Smith, MSN, RN

Deborah McCray Stewart, MSN, RN, FNP-C, CCHP

ANA Staff

Carol Bickford, PhD, RN-BC, CPHIMS — Content editor

Maureen Cones, Esq. — Legal counsel

Yvonne Humes, MSA — Project coordinator

Eric Wurzbacher, BA — Project editor

About the American Nurses Association

The American Nurses Association (ANA) is the only full-service professional organization representing the interests of the nation's 3.1 million registered nurses through its constituent and state nurses association and organizational affiliates. The ANA advances the nursing profession by fostering high standards of nursing practice, promoting the rights of nurses in the workplace, projecting a positive and realistic view of nursing, and by lobbying the Congress and regulatory agencies on healthcare issues affecting nurses and the public.

About Nursesbooks.org, The Publishing Program of ANA

Nursebooks.org publishes books on ANA core issues and programs, including ethics, leadership, quality, specialty practice, advanced practice, and the profession's enduring legacy. Best known for the foundational documents of the profession on nursing ethics, scope and standards of practice, and social policy, Nursebooks.org is the publisher for the professional, career-oriented nurse, reaching and serving nurse educators, administrators, managers and researchers, as well as staff nurses in the course of their professional development.

Scope of Correctional Nursing Practice

"Nursing is the protection, promotion, and optimization of health and abilities, prevention of illness and injury, alleviation of suffering through the diagnosis and treatment of human response, and advocacy in the care of individuals, families, communities, and populations" (ANA, 2010, p. 1). Nursing is both a science and an art, the essence of which is caring for and respecting human beings, including those in the correctional environment.

Correctional nursing is the protection, promotion, and optimization of health and abilities; prevention of illness and injury; alleviation of suffering through the diagnosis and treatment of human response; advocacy for and delivery of health care to individuals, families, communities, and populations under the jurisdiction of the criminal justice system.

Although the primary mission in correctional settings is to ensure the security and safety of inmates, staff, and the public, the primary role of nurses in correctional environments is, and has always been, the delivery of nursing care to inmates who are or may become patients. Within this environment, correctional nurses provide safe and competent nursing care, provide health education, and respond to and advocate for the health-care needs of patients. The term *inmate* is used throughout this specialty scope and standards document to identify the individual who is under the jurisdiction of the criminal justice system. The term *patient* identifies an inmate who is a consumer of healthcare services provided within the correctional system.

The History of Nurses within the Correctional Environment

The history of correctional nursing in America began as early as 1797 with the opening of New York City's Newgate Prison. Its warden, Thomas Eddy,

1

believed that criminals could be rehabilitated, and he established a school for the inmates as well as the first prison hospital and pharmacy.

During the 1800s, Dorothea Lynde Dix, a humanitarian, reformer, educator, crusader, and nurse best known for her strong advocacy for the mentally ill and prisoners, initiated reform in the prison setting (Reddi, 2005). She traveled throughout the country visiting prisons, meeting with wardens, and evaluating the various systems for effectiveness (Kokontis, 2007). Dorothea Dix described scenes of prisoners tied in chains, lying in their own filth with inadequate clothing, food, and light (Reddi, 2005). In 1845, Dix wrote "Remarks on Prisons and Prison Discipline in the United States" (Reddi, 2005). This work discussed the reforms she wanted the government to implement, including the education of prisoners and the separation of various types of offenders (Reddi, 2005). In spite of Dix's work, nursing remained unavailable in correctional facilities for quite some time. Instead, matrons, inmates, and corrections officers doled out inexpert medical care in dingy, unsanitary, and in most cases deplorable conditions (Sloan & Johnson, 2012).

November 1976 could be deemed the official start of the profession of correctional nursing (Schoenly, 2011). This was the date of the famous Supreme Court case *Estelle v. Gamble* (429 U.S. 97), which established health care as a constitutional right for U.S. inmates based on the Eighth Amendment (forbidding cruel and unusual punishment) (Schoenly, 2011). Correctional nursing began to gain increased visibility toward the end of the 20th century.

Rena Murtha, a pioneer in correctional nursing, described entering a large correctional facility where the nurse was perceived as a "tool of the warden, a slave of the physician and unknown to the patient" (1975). Since that time, correctional nursing practice has evolved into a variety of essential roles ranging from primary health care, mental health services, hospice, telemedicine, geriatrics, discharge planning, and chronic care management to management and administration. Today's correctional nurse is a valued and respected member of the correctional healthcare team.

Nursing in correctional settings is mentioned twice in the Institute of Medicine's report titled *The Future of Nursing: Leading Change, Advancing Health* (IOM, 2011). Both references make the point that nursing is diverse and that nurses will be present anywhere there are people who have healthcare needs. Dorothea Dix, Rena Murtha, and the nurses in correctional facilities today demonstrate passion, devotion, and advocacy in caring for an underserved and disenfranchised population that is, more often than not, forgotten by the public.

Health Care in Correctional Settings: A Brief Historical/Legal Perspective

Through most of the country's history, correctional settings in the United States provided little to no health care to inmates. As a result, inmate health outcomes were dismal. Courts rationalized the "hands-off" approach regarding correctional health care issues with (1) jurisdictional reasons and (2) respect for states' sovereignty to administer and operate correctional facilities within their borders. Thus, administrators in correctional settings had enormous freedom, with little regulation of, accountability for, or judicial oversight of daily operations that had an impact on inmates' health. The lack of self-regulation and judicial oversight spawned a rising number of prisoner petitions for relief from negative healthcare conditions of their confinement [*Coppinger v. Townsend*, 398 F.2d 392 (10th Cir. 1968); *Holt v. Sarver*, 442 F.2d 304 (8th Cir. 1971); *Martinez v. Mancusi*, 443 F.2d 921 (2d Cir. 1970); *Nelson v. Heyne*, 491 F.2d 352 (7th Cir. 1974); *Newman v. Alabama*, 349 F. Supp. 278 (M.D. Ala. 1972), *aff'd*, 503 F.2d 1320 (5th Cir. 1975)]; these forced courts to develop appropriate standards of judicial review for health care in correctional settings.

Finally, in 1976, the U.S. Supreme Court initiated development of the proper standards in the landmark case of *Estelle v. Gamble* (429 U.S. 97). Texas Department of Corrections inmate Gamble alleged that prison officials inflicted undue suffering on him when they failed to provide adequate health care for an injury he sustained in 1973 while incarcerated. The Supreme Court held that "deliberate indifference to serious medical needs of prisoners constitutes the 'unnecessary and wanton infliction of pain' . . . proscribed by the Eighth Amendment" (*Estelle*, 429 U.S. at 104). Thus, the *Estelle* decision gave judicial recognition to inmates' constitutional right to health care. *Estelle* also established a two-pronged national standard of judicial inquiry: (1) Did prison officials manifest "deliberate indifference" to offenders' medical needs?, and (2) Were those medical needs "serious"? (Posner, 1992). This national correctional healthcare inquiry standard applies whether the deliberate indifference is manifested by correctional healthcare providers in their responses to inmates' healthcare needs or by correctional officials who intentionally deny or delay access to health care or intentionally interfere with prescribed healthcare treatment (Blair, 2000).

The *Estelle* decision established the following Eighth Amendment constitutional rights for inmates related to health care:

■ The right to access care

■ The right to professional judgment

■ The right to prescribed healthcare treatment

Judicial inquiry utilizing the constitutional standard established in *Estelle v. Gamble* has led to positive restructuring of correctional healthcare systems throughout the United States. Development of case law and national standards on correctional health care have affirmed that prisoners are entitled to receive at least a minimally acceptable standard of health care (Blair, 2000). Nurses, the largest group of healthcare providers in the correctional setting, play a pivotal role in providing ethical care that meets acceptable minimum standards.

PREVALENCE OF CORRECTIONAL NURSES

The National Sample Survey of Registered Nurses, performed every four years by the Health Resources and Services Administration (HRSA), has reported on the number of nurses working in correctional settings since 2000. The most recent survey, completed in 2008, estimated that 20,772 registered nurses (0.8% of all registered nurses) reported that their primary employment setting was in a correctional facility (HRSA, 2010). The percentage of correctional nurses reported in 2008 remained unchanged from surveys completed in 2000 and 2004 (HRSA, 2000, 2004). The number of advanced practice registered nurses (APRNs) who provide clinical services within correctional settings remains unknown.

Correctional nurses, the American Nurses Association (ANA), and other stakeholders believe that the HRSA report underrepresents the number of nurses who work in correctional settings. First, the primary employer of a correctional nurse may be a university, county health department, private/for-profit ambulatory care agency, or home health organization that has been engaged to provide health care at a correctional facility. Second, the organizational unit may be a licensed hospital within a correctional system, or a hospital or clinic operated by the federal government that provides care for inmates or detainees. Third, many experienced correctional nurses have more than one employer, especially if they prefer a part-time or intermittent schedule.

No national organization regularly and reliably collects information on the number and characteristics of correctional nurses. Currently there is no accurate picture of the nursing workforce, despite a National Council of State

Boards of Nursing recommendation for standardizing the collection of these data. The National Forum of State Nursing Workforce Centers identifies correctional nursing in the National Nursing Workforce Minimum Datasets. If the recommended data sets are adopted by states, more data on correctional nursing will be available to describe the specialty.

Some consider correctional health care to be the last frontier of modern medicine, as the level of care given to those imprisoned can reflect the success of medicine, the effectiveness of legislation, the progress of nursing practice, and the advancement of society itself (Sloan & Johnson, 2012). As the correctional system grows and continues to evolve, correctional nurses will remain advocates to ensure that the patient is in an optimal state of physical and mental health to become a productive citizen upon return to the community.

POPULATION SERVED BY CORRECTIONAL NURSES

After three decades of soaring growth, incarceration rates in the United States have decreased. However, the United States continues to lead the world in rates of incarceration. At the end of 2009, 7.2 million people were on probation, parole, or in correctional facilities (Pew Center on the States, 2008).

The dramatic increases in the inmate population stem from policies aimed at punishing violations of parole and extending sentences, and from legislation requiring longer sentences. The war on drugs added to this explosive growth, with 73–83% of inmates reporting past drug use and 13–20% reporting injection drug use (Pew Center on the States, 2008;).

A view of the persons affected by imprisonment is disconcerting. Ethnic minorities are greatly overrepresented in correctional populations. African American males are incarcerated at rates nearly six times that of whites, and Hispanic males are incarcerated at nearly twice the rates of white males (Mauer & King, 2007).

The health needs of both adult and juvenile inmates are greater than they were a decade ago. The majority of the correctional population comes from disadvantaged backgrounds and socioeconomic groups associated with poverty and lack of access to regular healthcare services. Histories of excessive risky behaviors, trauma, alcohol and drug abuse, cigarette smoking, and poor diets prevail (Centers for Disease Control and Prevention [CDC], 2011). Not surprisingly, chronic diseases are also prevalent among these groups, with hypertension, diabetes, cardiovascular disease, obesity, and viral infections reported to be more common among inmates than the general population [Wilper et al., 2009; National Commission on Correctional Health Care (NCCHC), 2002; Binswanger, Krueger, & Steiner, 2009]. Additional challenges to healthcare delivery include lower literacy skills and educational attainment among inmates in correctional settings as compared to household populations (U.S. Department of Education, 1994).

Communicable diseases are of great concern in this country's often overcrowded and antiquated correctional facilities, because diseases are easily transmitted in these closed settings. The prevalence of human immunodeficiency virus (HIV), hepatitis C (HCV), hepatitis B (HBV), tuberculosis, and other infectious diseases is higher among inmates than in the general population (Hammett, 2006), a fact that presents challenges in the provision of care and discharge planning for the inmate who is a patient. Currently, it is estimated that approximately 150,000 HIV-positive persons are being released annually from U.S. correctional settings; these persons need reentry initiatives to prevent risky behaviors, obtain medications, and provide continuity of care (Rich et al., 2011).

Incarcerated persons represent the largest group to be infected with HCV in the United States, with an estimated prevalence of 12–35% as compared to 1–1.5% of the general population (CDC, 2012). It is becoming a leading cause of illness and death in some correctional settings (HCV Advocate, 2003).

Overcrowded and cramped quarters in correctional settings are also conducive to the rapid spread of other infectious diseases, such as influenza, scabies, and community-acquired methicillin-resistant *Staphylococcus aureus* (CA-MRSA) infections. There have been a number of CA-MRSA outbreaks in correctional settings among inmates after incarceration; these occurrences have prompted improvement in infection control practices and the development of treatment guidelines specific to prisons and jails to prevent disease spread (CDC, 2003; Malcolm, 2011).

Tuberculosis (TB) is particularly problematic for correctional facilities. The CDC (2006) indicates that the incidence of new TB cases among the U.S. population has remained at less than 10 cases per 100,000 persons since 1993, compared to substantially higher case rates reported in correctional populations. Latent TB infection (LTBI) prevalence among inmates may be as high as 25%.

Specialized populations, such as older adults, women, and juveniles, represent a smaller portion of the incarcerated population, but have unique characteristics that pose significant challenges to appropriate care in correctional facilities. Nevertheless, for some incarceration provides a window of opportunity to address health needs and improve health conditions.

The older-adult inmate cohort is increasing due to longer sentencing requirements (Pew Center on the States, 2008). This group suffers from age-related conditions earlier in life. Personal histories of poor nutrition, lack of preventive care, and high-risk behavior such as smoking and drug and alcohol use make a 50-year-old inmate's health status comparable to that of a 65-year-old living in the community (Smyer & Burbank, 2009). Related functional limitations, dementia, mobility deficits, incontinence, hearing and visual impairments, and chronic illnesses create special needs that are challenging for correctional settings to address, and often require nursing care and support that may not be necessary for other inmates. Frail elderly inmates may also be vulnerable to being preyed on by younger, stronger inmates (Loeb & AbuDagga, 2006).

Women are the fastest-growing segment of the correctional population. More than 200,000 women were in correctional settings, and more than 1 million were on parole in 2007, which represents an 800% increase over the past three decades (Pew Center on the States, 2008). Nearly two-thirds are incarcerated for nonviolent offenses, many of which are drug-related. The majority of incarcerated women are under the age of 35, with women of color being disproportionately represented. Histories of drug and alcohol abuse, sexual violence, trading sex for money or drugs, multiple sexual partners, sexually transmitted infections, and pregnancies in early adolescence put them at high risk for chronic and communicable diseases (Anno, 1997; Baral Abrams, Etkind, Burke, & Cram, 2008). Many are not married, do not have a high school education, and were unemployed before incarceration. Four percent are pregnant upon incarceration, and many of these pregnancies are classified as high risk [Women's Prison Association (WPA), 2009]. Incarcerated women are reported to have higher rates of diabetes, HIV, and sexually transmitted diseases, as well as higher rates of serious mental illnesses, drug abuse, depression, and other emotional problems in comparison to the male population. This results in female offenders using healthcare services more frequently than their male counterparts (Goldkuhle, 1999).

Juveniles confined to detention facilities are considered to be a high-risk group with many unmet developmental, medical, and mental health needs. Despite their youth, these individuals may present with one or more chronic illnesses, such as diabetes, asthma, seizure disorders, and learning and developmental disabilities. Approximately 11 million juveniles (under the age of 18 years) were arrested in 2008. Of those, 10% were referred to adult courts. Females make up about one-third of the juvenile arrests. As in the adult population, racial differences are evident, with the majority coming from impoverished backgrounds and single-parent households, with low levels of educational attainment, and histories of high risk-taking behaviors [Office of Juvenile Justice and Delinquency Programs (OJJDP), 2011]. Although their general health needs mirror those of their counterparts in the community, these youths have specific health problems resulting from their backgrounds and risky behaviors of violence, substance abuse, and sexual activity. Youths in confinement facilities have the highest rates of sexually transmitted infections (STIs) in the nation. Other health problems include traumatic injuries, significant dental needs, and higher pregnancy rates than their nonincarcerated peers (American Academy of Pediatrics, 2011). Suicide is a major public health concern among adolescents, in particular for those in confinement (American Academy of Pediatrics, 2011; Hayes, 2009).

Many inmates, including juveniles, are parents. In 2007, 65,600 women in custody reported being mothers, and 77% of these reported being the primary caretakers of their children (WPA, 2009). Incarceration results in abrupt separation from family, which can have a traumatic impact on the inmate's psychosocial and mental health during incarceration, and present challenges for the reestablishment of relationships when the inmate is released back to the community (Pew Center on the States, 2008).

Correctional settings have been dramatically affected by the deinstitutionalization of persons with mental illness in the community over the past decades; this trend has caused a tremendous increase in the numbers of inmates who have major psychiatric disorders. The new therapies, decreased insurance reimbursements, and tightened state and local healthcare budgets have resulted in decreased lengths of stay and a drastic reduction in the number of state and county mental hospitals and inpatient beds. Lack of available community financial and social system supports often results in persons with mental illness becoming nomads who eventually end up residing, in ever-increasing numbers, in America's correctional settings. The percentage of inmates with serious mental illnesses has nearly tripled in the past three decades. Estimates indicate that 16–20% of correctional populations are suffering from major psychiatric disorders and require mental health services (Fuller, Kennard, Eslinger, Lamb, & Pavle, 2010). Although many correctional facilities employ mental health staff, such as psychiatrists, psychologists, and other mental health workers, it is important for correctional nurses to build knowledge and skills that support nursing care for this population.

SETTINGS FOR CORRECTIONAL NURSING PRACTICE

Correctional health care takes place within juvenile confinement settings and adult correctional institutions (including jails and prisons). Correctional facilities vary widely in size and facility design, from large, multiple-facility systems to small, single facilities. Larger facilities may have observation beds, an infirmary, and skilled care and hospice beds, and may offer dialysis or other specialty services for this population. Persons under Department of Corrections (DOC) and criminal justice jurisdictions needing healthcare services may also be found in diversion, parole, probation, community halfway houses, specialty units within hospitals, joint mental health-DOC hospitals, and DOC-managed nursing homes.

There can be a wide variation in the number and skill mix of nurses employed in correctional facilities. The size and scope of health services provided have an impact on nurse staffing, as do facility configuration, patient acuity, and facility budgets. Larger systems may employ registered nurses (RNs) and advanced practice registered nurses (APRNs) with different educational levels and experience. Smaller and more rural areas tend to have lower staffing levels and some facilities staff with only one nurse. In addition to the initial challenges of attracting nurses to correctional settings, facilities located in rural areas and smaller facilities in nonmetropolitan areas may have difficulties with recruitment. Nevertheless, correctional nurses must ensure that appropriate nursing care is provided to patients in a timely manner by competent staff.

Nurses practicing in correctional systems must understand their responsibilities to the patients and larger correctional population. This involves delivery of nursing care to patients both in the health unit and on the tiers and pods where inmates are housed. Sometimes it becomes necessary for the nurse to provide immediate and urgent care in classrooms, dayrooms, or on the yard (outside where inmates exercise or where there is movement back and forth between facilities). The correctional nurse provides nursing care and treatment while demonstrating respect, caring, advocacy, and safety wherever the nurse encounters the patient.

Roles and Practice of the Correctional Nurse

Correctional nursing requires flexibility, attention to detail, critical thinking, a strong ability for clinical decision-making, and a sound grasp of the standards of professional practice. The nurse is often the primary or initial link to access to care for this population. The correctional nurse relies on comprehensive assessment and triage skills, as well as strong communication and negotiation skills. Utilization of the nursing process is critical to patient safety and good patient outcomes. Depending on the length of stay in a correctional facility, most inmates will require nursing services: some for treatment of minor illnesses or aliments, others for major health concerns needing appropriate follow-up. Correctional nurses have a primary role as patient advocates and champions for inmate health care.

PRIMARY CARE

Primary care is the model of care delivery in correctional settings for both juveniles and the adult population. The nurse's primary care role in this setting mirrors the role of the nurse in community, public health, and ambulatory care. Registered nurses and APRNs assume critical roles as the primary caregivers in the correctional setting and managers of the inmate's access to all other aspects of the healthcare system. Nurses usually are the first healthcare provider the patient encounters (Muse, 2009), and over the period of incarceration an inmate will see nurses more often than any other healthcare professional (Burrow, Knox, & Villanueva, 2006). Correctional nurses see patients upon arrival at the facility, every time the patient has a health concern, and whenever there is potential for injury or deterioration as a result of housing, work assignment, or an occurrence such as use of force. Nurses see patients for scheduled well-person and preventive care, in response to medical emergencies, and to deliver prescribed treatment. Nurses are responsible for ensuring continuity of care; thus, they see patients in chronic care clinics, make arrangements for inmates in advance of their release to the community, and resume care whenever an inmate returns to the facility. Therefore, correctional nurses in their primary role as caregiver have profound influence on the health, behavior, and well-being of incarcerated persons.

ACUTE CARE

The correctional nurse is usually the first healthcare responder to inmate or staff complaints of illness, emergencies, and trauma in the housing unit, recreation area, kitchen, or other location. The correctional nurse brings essential emergency equipment, performs a comprehensive assessment, and determines if the patient's condition warrants emergency treatment, including transport to the medical unit. If the nurse determines a life threatening condition exists, the emergency medical service (EMS) is activated either by the nurse or security staff. The correctional nurse directs the provision of first aid and basic life support to stabilize the patient until EMS arrives on the scene. If the illness or injury is not immediately life-threatening, the nurse will notify the physician and obtain orders for further management if necessary. The inmate/patient may be placed in the infirmary for twenty-four hour nursing care. Some correctional facilities have a full service correctional hospital to handle acute care issues or may contract for local community hospital services.

MEDICATION MANAGEMENT

In the correctional setting, a significant aspect of nursing practice involves medication administration and management. Correctional nurses are expected to have knowledge of the medications that are administered, which includes knowing the medication, appropriate dosage, side effects, contraindications, and food and drug interactions. Medication administration by correctional nurses must meet the same standard as medication administration in the community. Professional nurses must be knowledgeable with respect to their states' practice acts and statutes with regard to dispensing, administration, and delivery of prescription and other medications.

In some settings, established quantities of prescribed medications are delivered directly to the patient for self-administration. This type of administration is referred to as self-medication keep-on-person (SM-KOP). For patient safety, medications with a known history for potential abuse (e.g., prescription analgesics) and medications that have been associated with overdose (e.g., psychiatric medications) should be administered by direct observation (DO) or direct observed therapy (DOT). Facility procedures may permit delivery of medications by trained security staff to patients for self-administration.

Regardless of how patients receive their medications, the correctional nurse has a responsibility to ensure that patients know what medications they are taking and that they understand the dosage and possible side effects. In correctional systems where patients may use KOP medications, the nurse has a duty to assess the patient for competence to self-manage medications, including compliance with medication schedules and therapies. Finally, the correctional nurse is expected to work with trained custody staff and others to ensure that patients are able to receive their medications in a safe and timely manner.

HEALTH PROMOTION

Health promotion, maintenance, and education are of particular importance to the correctional population, because of limited healthcare access and poor prior lifestyle choices. Health promotion and surveillance require the skills of community health and public health nursing and play an important role in the healthcare management of this population, with a focus on quality assurance, prevention, and advocacy. Registered nurses as primary care providers in correctional settings provide health education and health promotion activities for healthy lifestyles, evaluate the effectiveness of planned care, encourage preventive health practices, and address public health issues.

Correctional nurses play an integral role in providing health education to inmates and correctional staff. Correctional nurses collaborate with other health-care providers and make best use of correctional resources to provide patient educa-tion aimed at helping inmates to engage in positive health and wellness behaviors.

In recent years, increasing attention has been given to the transition to commu-nity services following inmate release. This focus on transition to the community can have significant impact on recidivism and reentry. Correctional nurses play a critical role in establishing linkages to community healthcare resources so that inmates have an opportunity for continuity of care and a more successful return to society. The nurse's active role in discharge has different challenges for jails and prisons. Although reentry planning should start early during incarceration, those with shorter jail stays require more rapid attention to community transition than those with longer prison sentences. The longer prison time can allow time to build the health literacy and self-care skills that will enhance reentry success.

PRESERVATION OF SAFETY

There may be occasions when security concerns and the safety of the community may conflict with an individual patient's healthcare needs. Correctional nurses must be willing to effectively negotiate these dilemmas with security staff and/or administrative staff to resolve the conflict in a manner that preserves patient safety. Furthermore, the correctional environment requires that nurses carry out their practices in collaboration with security staff in order to maintain the strict safety orientation required in secure settings. Effective communication with security staff supports them in their mission of preserving safety and helps to strengthen nurses' voice in the correctional system. However, collaborating with security activities does not mean that correctional nurses should participate in security activities, which may include the collection of purely forensic evidence, body cavity searches, punitive disciplinary procedures, or the execution process (NCCHC, 2008).

Correctional systems exist to protect the public by preventing and controlling delinquency and crime. This is achieved by effective super-vision, rehabilitation, and meeting the basic human needs of offenders [American Corrections Association (ACA), 2002]. The prevailing feature experienced in the environment of a correctional facility is rigorous structure and accountability for people, objects, and processes in conformance to rules that ensure safety and security. Within the context of safe patient care, correctional nurses recognize that the promotion of patient and staff safety includes adherence to facility security rules and the provision of education to inmates and correctional staff about safe work practices and infection control measures. Correctional nurses understand that safe patient care is the right of all patients and the obligation of all healthcare staff (IOM, 2000). Although the inmate's right to health care is well established in state and federal law, the custody imperative of maintaining safety and security can create a challenge for nurses in delivering care that is consistent with professional standards of practice (Shelton, 2009; LaMarre, 2006).

One example of this challenge is that the custody environment limits the expression of caring that is fundamental to the nurse-patient relationship (Weiskopf, 2005). Common expressions of caring (touch, individualized attention, and empathic disclosure of personal information) are acknowledged in the literature as contributing to comfort, enhanced communication, and establishment of a therapeutic alliance with the patient—but are prohibited or extremely limited in the correctional setting (LaMarre, 2006; Weiskopf, 2005). Correctional nurses convey caring by placing emphasis on the interpersonal communication with the patient rather than physical or personal contact. Patient interactions that convey respect, are nonjudgmental, acknowledge the patient's subjective experience, are not rushed, and are in the genuine interest of the patient all express caring in the correctional setting (Weiskopf, 2005).

Another example is the ethical imperative to advocate for the patient when the patient's health or well-being may be compromised. Changes made by correctional systems to allow inmates self-care items, to create sheltered housing for vulnerable inmates, and to improve sanitation have been a result of nurses advocating for individual patients or for the health and well-being of the population as a whole. Other examples of advocacy include:

- Following up to ensure that patients who have scheduled appointments are escorted to the clinic.

- Ensuring that all requests for healthcare attention have been triaged appropriately by the end of the day,

- Reporting verbal or physical abuse.

- Collaborating with facility administrative staff, and elected and court officials to ensure inmates receive health services deemed necessary by qualified healthcare professionals, and that all legally sanctioned examinations are completed.

Collectively, advocacy by correctional nurses has resulted in sustained system improvement and improved conditions in correctional facilities (Weiskopf, 2005; LaMarre, 2006). Although correctional nurses may encounter difficulty when they advocate for their patients in the correctional setting, the provision of excellent patient assessment data and evidence-based nursing practices will support their nursing decisions.

SPECIAL CARE

Inmates in administrative or disciplinary confinement receive daily visits from the correctional nurse to collect medical requests and administer medication. Care is provided to the inmate either in a designated medical exam room near the housing area or in the medical unit. Death row inmates are directly observed by security with daily visits by the correctional nurse, chaplain and warden. The nurse delivers medication if prescribed, collects medical requests, and conducts sick calls if needed. Visits may be increased to every shift and as needed the week before execution.

CARE COORDINATION

Continuity of care in correctional environments is often interrupted by factors associated with security measures such as moves, restriction of movement, and limitation of personal items. Therefore, the correctional nurse provides critical care coordination services from the inmate's entry into the facility, through incarceration, and transition back into the community. Correctional nurses identify health issues, make appropriate referrals to advanced level and specialist providers, and ensure needed healthcare information is transmitted to all facilities that will provide health care to the inmate. An important correctional nurse responsibility includes coordination of health services in community settings needed during the inmate's incarceration and following discharge.

REQUISITE SKILLS AND KNOWLEDGE

Correctional nursing practice merges the knowledge and skills of many other nursing domains, including occupational health, emergency room, acute care, community health, psychiatric care, geriatrics, women's health, adolescent health, palliative, and end-of-life care (Shelton, 2009). Nurses assess, treat, and manage the care of patients with a variety of complex and often co-occurring health concerns. As the health needs of the population in correctional settings change, so too does the practice of nurses to meet those needs. For example, now that correctional facilities house three times more mentally ill individuals than all psychiatric facilities in the United States (Torrey, Kennard, Eslinger, Lamb, & Pavle, 2010), it is even more important that correctional nurses incorporate mental and emotional health, as well as physical health, considerations into every patient encounter.

Correctional nurses provide health care to their patients without regard to their criminal allegations, convictions, or histories. Under some circumstances, correctional nurses may therapeutically work with their patients to assist them in developing coping strategies when faced with anxiety related to upcoming court dates or pending release dates. Correctional nurses are expected to provide nursing care to their patients with compassion, empathy, commitment, competence, dedication, and a professional attitude.

Additional roles that correctional nurses fulfill include the provision of emergency services and health education to staff, visitors, and contractors who may be present in correctional facilities. Emergency services may include the provision of emergency first aid for minor injuries or illnesses onsite, or the provision of first aid and condition monitoring prior to transportation to a higher level of care for more serious health problems. Correctional nurses are often asked to provide education to correctional staff regarding common physical and mental health conditions seen in the correctional patient population, safe workplace practices, and basic first aid care that may be required of them during an emergency situation prior to the arrival of a medical staff member.

Finally, collaboration and problem-solving in this complex environment can take place only when each party understands and respects the work and interests of others (Weiskopf, 2005; Shelton, 2009; Shelton, Weiskopf, & Nicholson, 2010). Correctional nurses build and nurture the relationship with their custody colleagues. When nurses and correctional staff work collaboratively, the goals of custody and health care are additive rather than mutually exclusive.

Tenets of Correctional Nursing

1. NURSING PRACTICE IS INDIVIDUALIZED.

For the correctional setting, nursing practice respects diversity and is individualized to meet the needs of the patient, the patient's family, or the correctional population who is the focus of attention and to whom the professional registered nurse is providing health services in compliance with the state nurse practice act and regulations.

2. NURSES COORDINATE CARE BY ESTABLISHING PARTNERSHIPS.

The registered nurse establishes partnerships with persons, families, security personnel, and other providers, utilizing in-person and electronic communication, to reach a shared goal of delivering care. Because of the nature of the correctional environment, the correctional nurse must communicate with custody staff regarding family involvement or communication that has the potential to jeopardize security. The correctional nurse engages in collaborative interpersonal team planning based on mutual trust, respect, open discussion, and shared decision-making, recognizing the value and contributions of each team member.

3. CARING IS CENTRAL TO THE PRACTICE OF THE REGISTERED NURSE.

Although professional nursing promotes healing and health in a way that builds a relationship between nurse and patient, in the correctional setting the nurse must recognize security rules, therapeutic boundaries, and safety. Additionally, the correctional nurse promotes self-care and safety.

4. REGISTERED NURSES USE THE NURSING PROCESS TO PLAN AND PROVIDE INDIVIDUALIZED CARE TO THEIR PATIENTS.

Correctional nurses utilize theoretical and evidence-based knowledge of human experiences and responses to collaborate with patients to assess, diagnose, identify outcomes, plan, implement, and evaluate care. Nursing interventions are intended to produce beneficial effects, contribute to quality outcomes, and above all do no harm. Nurses evaluate the effectiveness of their care in relation to identified outcomes and use evidence-based practice to improve care (ANA, 2010). Critical thinking guides each step of the nursing process, problem solving, and decision-making.

5. A STRONG LINK EXISTS BETWEEN THE PROFESSIONAL WORK ENVIRONMENT AND THE REGISTERED NURSE'S ABILITY TO PROVIDE QUALITY HEALTH CARE AND ACHIEVE OPTIMAL OUTCOMES.

Regardless of the environment, correctional nurses have an ethical obligation to maintain and improve healthcare practices and foster a healthy work environment (ANA, 2001). Evidence suggests that negative, demoralizing, and unsafe conditions in the workplace contribute to medical errors, ineffective care delivery, and conflict and stress among health professionals. This is an important factor in patient safety, quality, care and treatment, best patient outcomes, advocacy, job satisfaction, recruitment, and retention. Correctional nurses must recognize that the obligations of their practice do not diminish or change because of the environment in which they practice.

Principles That Guide Correctional Nursing Practice

The following principles serve as the underpinnings for correctional nursing:

- Registered nurses' primary duties in the correctional setting are the prevention of illness, health promotion, health education, and restoration and maintenance of the health of patients in a spirit of compassion, concern, and professionalism.

- Nurses practice interprofessional collaboration with healthcare team members, correctional staff, and community colleagues (i.e., public health and/or specialty care professionals) to meet the holistic needs of patients, which include physical, psychosocial, and spiritual aspects of care.

- Nurses encourage each individual (patient, inmate, correctional staff, correctional nurse, and healthcare team member) to take responsibility for disease prevention and health promotion through education and self-care practices.

- Professionalism, compassion, care, and concern are displayed in every patient encounter.

- Each patient, regardless of circumstances, possesses intrinsic value and should be treated with dignity and respect.

- Patient confidentiality and privacy are respected and preserved at all times.

- Each patient receives quality care that is cost-effective and congruent with the latest evidence-based practice, scope and standards of practice, and clinical guidelines.

- In placing the patient at the center of care, the professional nurse must include the patient's family or significant other as part of the care continuum.

- Nursing leadership and management promote the highest quality of patient care through application of fair and equitable policies and procedures, with interprofessional collaboration with other healthcare team members and correctional staff.

- Nursing practice is guided by nurse administrators who foster professional and personal development; are sensitive to employee needs; give support, praise, and recognition; and encourage continuing education and participation in professional organizations.

■ Nurses are encouraged to contribute to generation of new correctional nursing knowledge through research activities, including dissemination of research findings.

Professional Nursing Ethics in the Correctional Setting

Code of Ethics for Nurses with Interpretive Statements (ANA, 2001) provides a framework for ethical nursing practice in the correctional setting. Although all nine provisions of the Code are applicable to correctional practice, several are of distinct importance due to the nature of the patient population and the characteristics of the practice environment. Note the following specific examples of the application of Provisions 1 through 9 in the correctional setting.

Provision 1. The nurse, in all professional relationships, practices with compassion and respect for the inherent dignity, worth, and uniqueness of every individual, unrestricted by considerations of social or economic status, personal attributes, or the nature of health problems.

In the largely punitive correctional environment, it is essential for nurses to encourage respect for the human dignity of inmates who are patients. An adequate nurse–patient relationship must be fostered without prejudice toward individuals who may be known to have committed heinous crimes or have great potential for violence. Providing nursing care in an environment controlled by criminal justice leadership can require strong patient advocacy to obtain the needed resources and provide necessary services to treat illness and improve health.

Provision 2. The nurse's primary commitment is to the patient, whether an individual, family, group, or community.

Primacy of the patient's interests can, at times, conflict with the primary importance of safety for staff and other inmates. Correctional nurses must be able to balance these competing interests in delivering health care in this setting. They may be called upon to advocate for patients in situations that could include coercion and potential abuse. In addition, given the nature of the correctional environment, nurses may be tempted to exert unnecessary power and control over the patient. This is neither a nursing role nor a therapeutic intervention.

Correctional nurses may be asked to participate in collecting medically based forensic evidence, such as body fluid samples, or to perform body cavity searches for security reasons. These actions negatively affect the nurse–patient relationship and violate the therapeutic nature of correctional nursing care.

The nurse–patient relationship is tempered by the firm application of professional boundaries in an environment where overfamiliarity and mixed motivations can alter traditional roles. The nurse must act in a manner that is in the best interest of the patient's health condition while maintaining a safe and secure environment. Those who cross professional boundaries place themselves, their peers, and others, including the patient, in a position of compromised security and personal safety.

Provision 3. *The nurse promotes, advocates for, and strives to protect the health, safety, and rights of the patient.*

The patient's right to privacy and the confidentiality of his or her medical information can also be challenged in the correctional setting. The fundamental trust between the nurse and patient can be breached by inappropriate communication of health conditions outside the healthcare team. Correctional nurses must be ever vigilant about providing information necessary to maintain safety and accomplish care requirements without excessive disclosure.

Provision 4. *The nurse is responsible and accountable for individual nursing practice and determines the appropriate delegation of tasks consistent with the nurse's obligation to provide optimum patient care.*

Responsibility and accountability for individual practice are major concerns for correctional nurses, who deliver care in an environment that may lack the support afforded to nurses working in other practice settings. For example, the increased autonomy required of many correctional nurses can blur scope-of-practice boundaries. Nurses working in the criminal justice system may not have a sound practice structure of well-established policies, procedures, guidelines, and job descriptions. They may be requested to perform inappropriate functions by uninformed or ill-advised colleagues. Correctional nurses must be able to clearly articulate their scope of practice, assert their moral obligations in these situations, and practice accordingly.

Provision 5. The nurse is responsible and accountable for individual nursing practice and determines the appropriate delegation of tasks consistent with the nurse's obligation to provide optimum patient care.

The unrelenting forces of the correctional environment can lead to significant moral distress. Correctional nurses rely on their moral self-respect to survive and thrive in a difficult care situation. Establishing a mechanism to deal with moral dilemmas in one's particular setting, developing a strong internal and external moral support system, and continuing development of moral competence are necessary components of a healthy and morally sound correctional nursing practice.

Provision 6. The nurse participates in establishing, maintaining, and improving healthcare environments and conditions of employment conducive to the provision of quality health care and consistent with the values of the profession through individual and collective action.

Nurses bring professional values to the environment in which they provide care, and therefore have opportunities to influence ethical practice in the correctional setting. Caring is a core nursing value and a part of a nurse's relationship with the patient, team members, correctional staff, and administration. Correctional nurses may face situations of competing values, loyalties, and obligations that generate tension and conflict. Satisfying solutions to these situations preserve the integrity of nursing values while accomplishing the goals of the institution.

Provision 7. The nurse participates in the advancement of the profession through contributions to practice, education, administration, and knowledge development.

Correctional nurses have an ethical obligation to advance the profession through knowledge development, dissemination, and application to practice. Specialty practice knowledge can be disseminated and applied through evidence-based practice guidelines and process improvement. This contributes to the ongoing development of the specialty's body of knowledge, advancing care for current and future patients.

Provision 8. The nurse collaborates with other health professionals and the public in promoting community, national, and international efforts to meet health needs.

With the majority of patients returning to the community, correctional nursing has a public health emphasis and therefore ethical responsibilities to the public. Reduction of communicable diseases and preventive disease practices improve the health of individual patients and the communities they return to upon release. Advocating for increased application of public health principles in the correctional setting is an important component of ethical correctional nursing practice.

Provision 9. The profession of nursing, as represented by associations and their members, is responsible for articulating nursing values, for maintaining the integrity of the profession and its practice, and for shaping social policy.

Correctional nurses do not practice in isolation from others in the profession of nursing; therefore, they have ethical responsibilities regarding participation in the larger nursing community. Maintaining contact and collaboration with the nursing community also allows opportunities to help shape a healthier society.

Correctional nurses may also find guidance in decision-making in the Code of Ethics established by the American Correctional Health Services Association (ACHSA), the Code of Ethics established by the American Corrections Association (ACA), and the position statement published by the International Council of Nursing (ICN) on the nurse's role in the care of detainees and prisoners.

In addition to ethical issues, care delivery and practice dilemmas may arise for the nurse and create challenges to the nurse's professional boundaries. Correctional nurses must incorporate insights from their professional nursing education, applicable nurse practice act and accompanying regulations, and professional scope of practice to address barriers that conflict with nursing practice, healthcare delivery, or requests for services. The correctional healthcare standards of the National Commission on Correctional Health Care and the American Correctional Association provide additional support to professional correctional nursing practice. It is possible to provide good care, demonstrate caring behaviors, and support and advocate for patients without violating correctional policies and rules.

Correctional Registered Nurses

The correctional registered nurse is expected to demonstrate professional nursing practice, proficient use of the nursing process, clinical expertise, competence, knowledge of quality improvement measures, evidence-based research, leadership and management, and critical and systems thinking. In addition, the professional nurse will demonstrate integrity, nursing values, ethical principles, and moral practices. Correctional nurses play an important role in developing, directing, and guiding other members of the health team and in advancing the profession of nursing. The registered nurse is responsible for overseeing the delivery of health care. When the nursing care team is composed of a variety of licensed and unlicensed staff members, the registered nurse assumes leadership responsibilities for other staff members.

Knowledge and skills in delegation and communication are important areas of expertise for the professional nurse. Traditionally, little focus has been placed on the leadership and clinical roles of nurses in correctional settings. An understanding of the scope of practice for each licensed staff member and the skill level and job requirements of unlicensed personnel are of particular importance in the correctional setting, where the complexity of patient health needs, concerns for patient safety, fiscal accountability, and concerns about access to patient care can be numerous.

Registered nurses practicing in correctional settings must have knowledge of the criminal justice system, an understanding of the process of litigation, legal aspects of nursing practice, constitutional rights of this population, and possible litigation that may be present in their respective institutions. This additional knowledge assists nurses in understanding and managing their practice in this setting.

Advanced Practice Registered Nurses in the Correctional Setting

The advanced practice registered nurse (APRN) roles include those of clinical nurse specialist (CNS), certified nurse practitioner (CNP), certified midwife (CNM), and certified registered nurse anesthetist (CRNA). Increasingly, correctional institutions are recognizing the value of APRNs to effective care delivery. The APRN's practice is characterized by a depth and breadth of knowledge in nursing practice, as well as in specific specialty practice areas. This clinician demonstrates an advanced understanding of nursing and advanced skills in diagnosis and treatment, as well as care delivery. The APRN has the ability to incorporate knowledge of the correctional health field in planning, implementing, and managing evidence-based health care.

In collaboration with the designated nurse leader, the APRN is expected to participate in guiding the practice and critical thinking of nursing and other healthcare personnel, carry out advanced clinical practice activities, manage one or more clinical practice settings, incorporate scientific knowledge from other disciplines into practice and management, and evaluate the health care provided in those settings through a comprehensive quality improvement system. In the correctional environment, the CNS, CNP, or CNM with prescriptive authority may serve as the sole primary care provider. The CNS and CNP may also serve in the clinical educator role. The APRN should play an important role in the development, role modeling, and coaching of other professional nurses and in enhancing professional nursing practice in the correctional setting.

Executive Nurse Leadership in the Correctional Setting

The role of the executive nurse leader in the correctional setting is instrumental to safe nursing practice and quality patient care delivery. This individual plays a critical role in creating a healthy work environment, articulating standards of practice, giving a voice to nurses and nursing, and working with other senior colleagues to enhance the delivery of health care.

Graduate nursing education at the master's and doctoral level best prepares the correctional nurse to function in administrative roles such as chief nursing officer or health service administrator for large systems. Even in smaller systems, the successful nurse leader should be prepared at the master's level. Clinical expertise, knowledge of research and evidence-based practice, systems thinking, and quality models, combined with their administrative and leadership skills, as well as management experience, give these nurse leaders the depth and breadth of preparation to serve at the senior executive level. This level of educational preparation further prepares them to address the fiscal management responsibilities, inherent political and organizational complexities, and policy issues of the correctional healthcare delivery system. The senior executive nurse leader is additionally prepared for the public relations aspects of leading and championing the health and staffing needs of the correctional healthcare facility.

Educational Preparation for Correctional Nurses

The preferred educational preparation for the registered nurse for entry into correctional nursing is at the baccalaureate level. This level of entry has increased importance given the complexity of patient needs and the level of decision-making and autonomy of practice in this setting. Continuing professional development is expected and necessary, as care delivery and requisite expertise expand into many specialty areas. Correctional nurses and leaders in correctional health care are encouraged to promote further education at the baccalaureate or graduate levels.

Correctional nursing curriculum content and associated clinical practicum experiences are rarely incorporated into formal academic programs at the undergraduate nursing level. If such experiences are included, they most often consist of invited guest speakers addressing care of such vulnerable populations during community health courses. Similarly, a paucity of specific correctional nursing content and specialty practice opportunities characterizes graduate-level educational programs, especially for those preparing registered nurses for the advanced practice roles of clinical nurse specialist, certified nurse practitioner, and certified nurse midwife. Some academic nursing programs have initiated discussions about strategies to formally integrate correctional nursing content or tracks within existing or future curricula. Some colleges offer a correctional nursing certificate, which may be obtained in the college setting or through online course completion. Intern and extern programs available in some correctional settings allow the interns/externs to work with inmates who have a variety of physical ailments and impairments. The intern/externs may also care for incarcerated patients who suffer from a wide array of mental disorders, ranging from serious, chronic mental illness and progressive disorders to transient, crisis-based disturbances.

Depending on the correctional setting of interest, correctional nurses may elect to expand their skills and knowledge in clinical specialty programs such as pediatric, psychiatric–mental health, oncology, hospice and palliative care, or gerontological nursing. Formal preparation for nursing administration roles may be achieved through completion of a graduate-level program in nursing administration. Others may elect to seek advanced degrees in business administration, economics, finance, or law to complement their nursing education preparation and experience. These graduate-level-prepared correctional nurses are expected to demonstrate additional competencies beyond those of the correctional registered nurse.

Nurses interested in the correctional environment may find additional learning opportunities available in college-level criminal justice courses and continuing education and certificate programs offered by such organizations as the American Correctional Association and National Commission on Correctional Health Care.

Specialty Certification in Correctional Nursing

Certification and advanced certification in correctional health are available through the National Commission on Correctional Health Care, the American Correctional Association, and the American Nurses Credentialing Center (ANCC).

The NCCHC identifies three types of certification. The Certified Correctional Health Professional (CCHP) certification was established in 1991. The CCHP designation identifies the individual as one who has demonstrated mastery of national standards and the knowledge expected of leaders working in the field of correctional health care. CCHP-A for the advanced level was established in 1994. It is designed to assess experience in and knowledge of the delivery of healthcare services in correctional environments. CCHP-RN for the registered nurse, established in 2010, provides formal recognition of nurses' specialized knowledge, skills, and experience specific to the practice of nursing in correctional settings. Whereas nursing licensure establishes legal authority for an individual to practice nursing, specialty certification reflects achievement of the special knowledge and skills needed for a particular practice area.

In 2007, the ACA established its own certification program for correctional nurses. ACA's Corrections Certification Program is offered in two specialty categories. The Certified Corrections Nurse Manager (CCN/M) certification category includes individuals who work as nurse managers in a correctional environment. They are management staff who may contribute to the development of policy and procedures, are responsible for the implementation of those policies and procedures, and have authority over staff members. The Certified Corrections Nurse (CCN) category is composed of staff nurses who work in correctional environments with staff and offenders. This designation includes those responsible for implementing agency policies and procedures.

Certification programs often require proof of ongoing continuing education, which is available through online learning opportunities; attending conferences; and reading journals, articles, and other educational materials.

Certification in nursing administration and other nursing specialties is available through ANCC and other certification bodies. Other practice certification and credentialing processes, such as ACLS, TNCC, CDE (Certified Diabetes Educator), CCRN (Critical Care Registered Nurse certification), and the like, may also be recommended or required for specific correctional settings.

Trends and Issues in Correctional Nursing

Primary care must be provided efficiently, effectively, and equitably to the entire correctional population. The many barriers to the establishment of an adequate correctional healthcare delivery system have included:

- The poor health status of the correctional system population

- The volume of healthcare services utilized

- Conflicts with security

- The living environment of correctional facilities and its association with hypertension, aggression, increased endocrine arousal, increased transmission of infectious disease, depression, and violence (Anno, 2001)

With the advent of accreditation by the NCCHC, The Joint Commission (TJC) and the ACA developed guidelines that describe the organization of an adequate delivery system of correctional health care. Also with accreditation came certification programs in correctional health care developed by the ACA, ANA, and the NCCHC. Educational programs and conferences on salient topics in correctional health care were developed and correctional health professionals recognized that they were now a certified specialty with their own body of knowledge distinct to the environment in which they worked.

Professional organizations emerged, such as the Academy of Correctional Health Professionals and the American Correctional Health Services Association, which led to an exchange of ideas among professionals working in similar environments, creating a support system among the providers.

In the early 1970s, the very few published articles related to correctional health care were descriptive studies on the needs of the incarcerated or an individual's experience in working in a correctional institution. As the correctional healthcare domain developed, literature and publications on best practices and research relating to correctional health care increased.

In 2010, the Robert Wood Johnson Foundation (RWJF) and the Institute of Medicine (IOM) jointly released *The Future of Nursing: Leading Change, Advancing Health,* calling it a blueprint for transforming the American health system by strengthening nursing care and better preparation of nurses to help lead reform. This report calls for increasing the percentage of nurses holding the bachelor of science degree (BSN) or higher and for doubling the number of doctorate holders by 2020. The report indicates that these changes will require new competency-based curricula, seamless educational progression, more funding for accelerated programs, student diversity, and stronger employer incentives to spur progression (IOM, 2011).

Due to changes in the patient population within the correctional system, nurses can anticipate enormous challenges in the provision of health care. Older and sicker patients, expanding demands for health care, more complex technology, and new healthcare settings and team configurations are all emerging as the country struggles to overcome the nursing shortage and implement the Affordable Care Act (Cardwell & Gilmore, 2011).

The United States incarcerates a higher share of its population than any other country in the world. Even though the rate of incarceration has dropped in the past five years, expenditures for correctional health care have not decreased [Bureau of Justice Statistics (BJS), 2011]. The aging of the correctional system population can be attributed to what some have called a "perfect storm," fueled by tough-on-crime legislation that mandates harsher sentencing and curtails the powers of judges with elimination of parole. With years of increased sentencing, the U.S. correctional system is saddled with a booming elderly and chronically ill population (Gibbons & Katzenbach, 2006).

High rates of disease and illness among this patient population, coupled with inadequate funding for correctional health care, endanger patients, staff, and the public. Much of the public dismisses jails and prisons as sealed institutions where what happens inside remains inside. In the context of diseases and illnesses that naturally travel from one environment into another, that view is short-sighted. Left untreated, staph infections, and other infectious diseases such as tuberculosis, hepatitis C, and AIDS, directly affect families, neighborhoods, and communities (Gibbons & Katzenbach, 2006).

The correctional patient population has a disproportionate number of Hispanics and African Americans (BJS, 2011). For this reason, medical and mental health programs must be established with an eye toward cultural diversity. Cultural diversity encompasses gender, disability, sexual identity, residency, geographic location, socioeconomic status, religion, age, family dynamics, and a host of other factors. Taking the time to identify these factors and incorporating them into a plan of care is the first step in establishing multicultural awareness. Considering the IOM report findings, colleges and employers of correctional health program graduates should seek more individuals who are able to cross cultural barriers and identify with their population in planning and delivering those patients' health care (Lasko, 2012).

As a result of poverty, substance abuse, and years of poor health care, correctional patients as a group are much less healthy than the average

American citizen. Every year 1.5 million people are released from jails and prisons, at least 350,000 of whom have a serious mental illness (BJS, 2011). Protecting public health and safety, reducing human suffering, and limiting the financial costs of untreated illness that causes recidivism all depend on adequate discharge planning and reentry programs. The high rate of recidivism among offenders suggests that current correctional system programs have not been useful and that discharge planning has not been effective.

According to an IOM (2010) report, the "silo" approach of single-provider management must soon give way if we are to meet future healthcare challenges. Correctional facilities have a tremendous opportunity to improve the care provided inside the correctional facility/institution and protect the public health of the nation. The following suggested actions address the improvement of health care in the correctional environment:

- **Partner with health providers from the community**. Seamless collaboration among departments of corrections, detention centers, and health providers from the community, working together on common projects for delivering high-quality health care (i.e., adopting a public health model of health care), brings success in treating diseases and creating effective discharge plans.

- **Build partnerships within facilities**. Correctional healthcare staff must build collaborative relationships with correctional administrators and officers so that the requirements of special-needs patients can be addressed in a team approach.

- **Commit to caring for patients with mental illness**. Commitment by legislatures and executive branch officials of adequate resources for identifying and treating mental illness while the patient is incarcerated and upon release is critical. Too often, patients with co-occurring substance abuse and mental illness are refused entry into programs for substance abuse, and vice versa. Paying for community-based services will not eliminate criminal justice involvement among some portion of the released patients with severe mental illness. Nevertheless, failure to invest in appropriate reentry services only compounds the problems, increasing the costs to society and causing additional pain and suffering to the individuals involved.

- **Screen, test, and treat for infectious disease**. Screening tests and treatment of infectious diseases in every U.S. prison and jail, in collaboration with the public health department and in compliance with national guidelines, helps ensure continuity of care while persons are incarcerated and upon their release.

■ **Extend Medicare and Medicaid services to eligible patients** so that correctional facilities can receive federal funding to help provide correctional health care. Until Congress is able to enact such legislation, states should ensure that benefits are available to patients upon release.

NEW TECHNOLOGY

The application of new technology, such as telehealth, and now electronic medical records (EMRs), is crucial if coordination of health care and continuity of care are to be attained. The utilization of telehealth for specialist appointments has increased public safety and decreased the need for officer transport by decreasing the movement of patients outside of the correctional facility. Telehealth has made specialist care more accessible and provides more timely consults. Telehealth can also eliminate appointments at physicians' offices and benefit facilities without 24/7 healthcare coverage. Call centers designed to provide adjunct nursing or mental health staff can provide a much-needed service to facilities without continuous on-site care (Kesler, 2012).

Today's healthcare industry is faced with increasing demand for information related to the financial, clinical, administrative, and managed care aspects of healthcare delivery. With this in mind, correctional healthcare organizations recognize that they must implement advanced technology to meet the complex demands of other healthcare agencies, professional associations, accrediting bodies, managed care groups, and insurance groups. The use of an electronic medical record ensures that information is transferred in a timely manner, confidentiality is maintained, and accurate data are available (Knight, 2009). There are now multiple software companies that have developed EMR technology specific to correctional health care. Correctional nurses should work with these companies to develop guidelines, protocols, and processes that are specific to the management of common patient conditions and scheduling processes.

ADMINISTRATIVE SEGREGATION

Administrative segregation, while generally a security concern, has received a great deal of attention from documentaries, news reporters, and mental health professionals. The increasing use of high-security segregation is often seen as counterproductive, causing violence inside the facility and contributing to violence after release. Separating dangerous or vulnerable inmates from the general population is, however, part of managing a safe correctional facility. In some systems around the country, the push for public safety, coupled with the public demand for tough punishment, has had serious adverse effects, such as inmate patients locked up in their cells for 23 hours per day with little opportunity to be productive or prepared for their release.

Patients should be carefully screened for mental health problems. Meaningful contact should be made so that patients are free from extreme physical and mental health deterioration that causes lasting harm. Patients with mental illness that would make them particularly vulnerable to damage from the conditions in segregation should be housed in secure therapeutic units. Finally, to the extent that safety allows, patients should be provided the opportunity to fully engage in treatment, work, study, and other activities.

COLLABORATION AND ENTREPRENEURSHIP

Many healthcare systems outside the correctional environment are gearing up for the collaborative challenge issued by the IOM. Nurse entrepreneurs have developed managed care companies to provide health care in correctional settings. These nurses have been very successful in obtaining public offerings and receiving enhanced capital for expansion of their corporations. Nursing entrepreneurs realize that without control of the budget for correctional health care, few changes can be made in the management of the correctional healthcare system. Private-sector healthcare companies have the ability to negotiate lower hospitalization rates, utilize emergency rooms less, and offer a higher level of job placement that provides a recruitment-incentive advantage over other systems. These programs, which are designed to specialize in correctional health care, can offer clinical guidelines, education, accreditation, and attractive career patterns.

Summary of the Scope of Correctional Nursing Practice

Correctional nurses must be advocates for their patients by maintaining adequate healthcare systems, following accreditation guidelines, and maintaining continuing education specific to the changing and challenging needs of the correctional population. Correctional nurses must develop strong interprofessional collaborative models to evolve this specialty practice.

Providing health care to an underserved population in a challenging environment requires personal and professional commitment and a high degree of cultural sensitivity. Collecting, measuring, and analyzing statistical data to more efficiently manage the systems and processes used to deliver health care is not a luxury, but rather a necessary management tool. Nurse managers must rely on more than intuition, past experience, inadequate data, and anecdotal information. Knowledge-based management can be applied at any facility if it is done with the recognition that each facility has different needs. Although the process of measuring, evaluating, and adjusting procedures may seem daunting, in reality it provides the efficient measures necessary for correctional facilities to keep pace with a changing environment.

> *Knowledge is not enough: we must apply*
>
> *Willing is not enough, we must do*
>
> —Goethe*

* Von Goethe, J. W. Retrieved from www.brainyquote.com/quotes/authors/j /johann_wolfgang_von_goeth.html

Standards of Correctional Nursing Practice

Significance of the Standards

The Standards of Correctional Nursing Practice are authoritative statements of the duties that all registered nurses, regardless of role, population, or specialty, are expected to perform competently. The standards published herein may be utilized as evidence of the standard of care, with the understanding that application of the standards is context dependent. The standards are subject to change with the dynamics of the nursing profession, as new patterns of professional practice are developed and accepted by the nursing profession and the public. In addition, specific conditions and clinical circumstances may also affect the application of the standards at a given time (e.g., during a natural or man-made disaster). The standards are subject to formal, periodic review and revision.

The competencies that accompany each standard may be evidence of compliance with the corresponding standard. The list of competencies is not exhaustive. Whether a particular standard or competency applies depends on the circumstances.

Standards of Practice for Correctional Nursing

Standard 1. Assessment

The correctional registered nurse collects comprehensive data pertinent to the patient's health and/or the situation.

COMPETENCIES
The correctional registered nurse:

■ Collects comprehensive and holistic data, including, but not limited to, physical, functional, psychosocial, emotional, cognitive, sexual, cultural, age-related, environmental, spiritual/transpersonal, and economic assessments, in a systematic and ongoing process while acknowledging the uniqueness of the person.

■ Elicits the patient's values, preferences, expressed needs, and knowledge of the healthcare situation to utilize such information as appropriate within the context of the correctional setting.

■ Involves the patient, family, correctional staff, and other healthcare providers, as appropriate, in holistic data collection.

■ Identifies barriers (e.g., psychosocial, literacy, financial, cultural) to effective communication and makes appropriate adaptations.

■ Recognizes the impact of personal attitudes, values, and beliefs on the patient's health status.

■ Assesses the impact of family dynamics on the patient's health and wellness.

■ Prioritizes data collection based on the patient's immediate condition, or the anticipated needs of the patient or situation.

■ Uses appropriate evidence-based assessment techniques, instruments, and tools.

■ Synthesizes available data, information, and knowledge relevant to the situation to identify patterns and variances.

- Applies ethical, legal, and privacy guidelines and policies to the collection, maintenance, use, and dissemination of data and information.

- Recognizes patients as the authority on their own health by identifying their care preferences.

- Documents relevant data in a retrievable format.

ADDITIONAL COMPETENCIES FOR THE GRADUATE-LEVEL-PREPARED CORRECTIONAL NURSE AND THE APRN

The graduate-level-prepared correctional nurse or advanced practice registered nurse:

- Initiates and interprets diagnostic tests and procedures relevant to the patient's current status.

- Assesses the effect of interactions among individuals, family, community, and social systems on health and illness.

Standard 2. Diagnosis

The correctional registered nurse analyzes the assessment data to determine the diagnoses, health concerns, or organizational issues.

COMPETENCIES

The correctional registered nurse:

- Derives the diagnoses, health concerns, or organizational issues from assessment data.

- Validates the diagnoses, health concerns, or organizational issues with the patient, family, and other healthcare providers when possible and appropriate.

- Identifies actual or potential risks to the patient's health and safety or barriers to health; these may include, but are not limited to, interpersonal, systematic, or environmental circumstances.

- Uses standardized classification systems and clinical decision support tools, when available, in identifying diagnoses.

- Documents the diagnoses, health concerns, or organizational issues in a manner that facilitates determination of the expected outcomes and plan.

ADDITIONAL COMPETENCIES FOR THE GRADUATE-LEVEL-PREPARED CORRECTIONAL NURSE AND THE APRN

The graduate-level-prepared correctional nurse or advanced practice registered nurse:

- Systematically compares and contrasts clinical findings with normal and abnormal variations and developmental events in formulating differential diagnoses.

- Utilizes complex data and information obtained during interview, examination, and diagnostic processes in identifying diagnoses.

- Assists staff in developing and maintaining competence in the diagnostic process.

Standard 3. Outcomes Identification

The correctional registered nurse identifies expected outcomes for a plan individualized to the patient or the situation.

COMPETENCIES

The correctional registered nurse:

- Involves the patient, family, healthcare and community providers, correctional personnel, and others in formulating expected outcomes when possible and appropriate.

- Derives culturally appropriate expected outcomes from the diagnoses.

- Considers associated risks, security issues, benefits, costs, current scientific evidence, expected trajectory of the condition, and clinical expertise when formulating expected outcomes.

- Defines expected outcomes in terms of the patient, patient culture, values, ethical considerations, environment, and situation while considering associated risks, security issues, benefits and costs, and current scientific evidence.

- Includes a time estimate for attainment of expected outcomes.

- Develops expected outcomes that provide direction for continuity of care.

- Modifies expected outcomes according to changes in the patient's status or evaluation of the situation.

- Documents expected outcomes as measurable goals.

ADDITIONAL COMPETENCIES FOR THE GRADUATE-LEVEL-PREPARED CORRECTIONAL NURSE AND THE APRN

The graduate-level-prepared correctional nurse or advanced practice registered nurse:

- Identifies expected outcomes that incorporate scientific evidence and are achievable through implementation of evidence-based practices.

- Identifies expected outcomes that incorporate cost and clinical effectiveness, patient satisfaction, and continuity and consistency among providers.

- Differentiates outcomes that require care process interventions from those that require system-level interventions.

Standard 4. Planning

The correctional registered nurse develops a plan that prescribes strategies and alternatives to attain expected outcomes.

COMPETENCIES

The correctional registered nurse:

- Develops an individualized plan in partnership with the patient, family, and others considering the patient's characteristics or situation, including but not limited to values, beliefs, spiritual and health practices preferences, choices, developmental level, coping style, culture and environment, safety, and available technology.

- Establishes the plan priorities with the patient, family, correctional personnel, and others as appropriate.

- Includes strategies in the plan to address each of the identified diagnoses or issues. These may include, but are not limited to, strategies for:

  - Promotion and restoration of health;

  - Prevention of illness, injury, and disease;

  - The alleviation of suffering; and

  - Supportive care for those who are dying.

- Includes strategies for health and wholeness across the lifespan.

- Provides for continuity of care in the plan.

- Incorporates an implementation pathway or timeline in the plan.

- Utilizes the plan to provide direction to other members of the health-care team and correctional personnel.

- Defines the plan to reflect current statutes, rules and regulations, guidelines, and standards.

- Considers the economic impact of the plan on the patient, family, caregivers, or other affected parties.

- Explores practice settings and safe space and time for the correctional nurse and patient to explore suggested, potential, and alternative options.

■ Modifies the plan according to the ongoing assessment of the patient's response and other outcome indicators.

■ Documents the plan in a manner that uses standardized language or recognized terminology.

ADDITIONAL COMPETENCIES FOR THE GRADUATE-LEVEL-PREPARED CORRECTIONAL NURSE AND THE APRN

The graduate-level-prepared correctional nurse or advanced practice registered nurse:

■ Identifies assessment strategies, diagnostic strategies, and therapeutic interventions that reflect current evidence, including data, research, literature, and expert clinical knowledge.

■ Selects or designs strategies to meet the multifaceted needs of complex patients.

■ Includes the synthesis of the patient's values and beliefs regarding nursing and medical therapies in the plan.

■ Leads the design and development of the interprofessional processes to address the identified diagnosis or issue.

■ Actively participates in the development and continuous improvement of systems that support the planning process.

Standard 5. Implementation

The correctional registered nurse implements the identified plan.

COMPETENCIES

The correctional registered nurse:

- Partners with the patient, family, significant others, caregivers, and correctional personnel as appropriate to implement the plan in a safe, realistic, and timely manner.

- Demonstrates caring behaviors toward patients, their families, significant others, and others receiving or inquiring about care.

- Utilizes technology to measure, record, and retrieve patient data; implement the nursing process; and enhance nursing practice.

- Utilizes evidence-based interventions and treatments specific to the diagnosis or problem.

- Provides holistic care that addresses the needs of diverse populations across their lifespan.

- Advocates for health care that is sensitive to the needs of patients, with particular emphasis on the needs of diverse populations.

- Applies appropriate knowledge of major health problems and cultural diversity in implementing the plan of care.

- Applies available healthcare technologies to maximize access and optimize outcomes for patients.

- Utilizes resources and systems of the correctional facility and within the community to implement the plan.

- Collaborates with nursing colleagues, healthcare providers, correctional personnel, and others from diverse backgrounds to implement and integrate the plan.

- Accommodates different styles of communication used by patients, families, significant others, other caregivers, correctional personnel, and healthcare providers.

- Integrates traditional and complementary healthcare practices as appropriate.

- Implements the plan in a timely manner in accordance with patient safety goals and consistent with correctional practices that promote the safety of the community.

- Promotes the patient's capacity for the optimal level of participation and problem solving.

- Documents implementation and any modifications, including changes or omissions, of the identified plan.

ADDITIONAL COMPETENCIES FOR THE GRADUATE-LEVEL-PREPARED CORRECTIONAL NURSE AND THE APRN

The graduate-level-prepared correctional nurse or advanced practice registered nurse:

- Facilitates utilization of systems, organizations, and community resources to implement the plan.

- Supports collaboration with nursing, other healthcare colleagues, and correctional personnel to implement the plan.

- Incorporates new knowledge and strategies to initiate change in nursing care practices if desired outcomes are not achieved.

- Assumes responsibility for safe and efficient implementation of the plan.

- Uses advanced communication skills to promote relationships between nurses and patients, to provide a context for open discussion of the patient's experiences, and to improve patient outcomes.

- Actively participates in the development and continuous improvement of systems that support implementation of the plan.

Standard 5A. Coordination of Care

The correctional registered nurse coordinates care delivery.

COMPETENCIES

The correctional registered nurse:

- Organizes the components of the plan, especially those related to safety and transitions of care.

- Manages the patient's care so as to maximize independence and quality of life considering the constraints of confinement.

- Assists the patient to identify options for alternative care.

- Communicates with the patient, family, community healthcare professionals, and healthcare and correctional systems during transitions in care.

- Advocates for the delivery of dignified and humane care by the interprofessional team.

- Completes arrangements or referrals to APRNs, physicians, behavioral health providers, and/or other facility healthcare providers as appropriate.

- Makes arrangements or referrals for follow-up services with community clinicians.

- Documents the coordination of care.

ADDITIONAL COMPETENCIES FOR THE GRADUATE-LEVEL-PREPARED CORRECTIONAL NURSE AND THE APRN

The graduate-level-prepared correctional nurse or advanced practice registered nurse:

- Provides leadership in the coordination of interprofessional health care for integrated delivery of patient care services.

- Synthesizes data and information to prescribe necessary system and community support measures, including modifications of surroundings.

Standard 5B. Health Teaching and Health Promotion

The correctional registered nurse employs strategies to promote health and a safe environment.

COMPETENCIES
The correctional registered nurse:

- Provides health teaching that addresses such topics as healthy lifestyles, risk-reducing behaviors, developmental needs, activities of daily living, and preventive self-care.

- Uses health promotion and health teaching methods appropriate to the situation and the patient's values, beliefs, health practices, developmental level, learning needs, readiness and ability to learn, language preference, spirituality, culture, and socioeconomic status.

- Provides educational material on a variety of health topics in areas accessible to all patients (e.g., housing area, library).

- Seeks opportunities for feedback and evaluation of the effectiveness of the strategies used.

- Uses information technologies to communicate health promotion and disease prevention information to the patient in a variety of settings.

- Provides patients with information about intended effects and potential adverse effects of therapies and medications.

ADDITIONAL COMPETENCIES FOR THE GRADUATE-LEVEL-PREPARED CORRECTIONAL NURSE AND THE APRN
The graduate-level-prepared correctional nurse or advanced practice registered nurse:

- Synthesizes empirical evidence on risk behaviors, learning theories, behavioral change theories, motivational theories, epidemiology, and other related theories and frameworks when designing health education information and programs.

- Conducts personalized health teaching and counseling while considering comparative effectiveness research recommendations.

■ Designs health information and patient education appropriate to the patient's developmental level, learning needs, readiness to learn, and cultural values and beliefs.

■ Evaluates health information resources, such as the Internet, in the area of practice for accuracy, readability, and comprehensibility to help patients access quality health information.

■ Engages consumer alliances and advocacy groups, as appropriate, in health teaching and health promotion activities.

■ Provides anticipatory guidance to individuals, families, groups, and communities to promote health and prevent or reduce the risk of health problems.

Standard 5C. Consultation

The graduate-level-prepared specialty nurse or advanced practice registered nurse provides consultation to influence the identified plan, enhance the abilities of others, and effect change.

**COMPETENCIES FOR THE GRADUATE-LEVEL
PREPARED CORRECTIONAL NURSE AND THE APRN**

The graduate-level-prepared correctional nurse or advanced practice registered nurse:

- Synthesizes clinical data, theoretical frameworks, and evidence when providing consultation.

- Facilitates the effectiveness of a consultation by involving the patient, family, significant others, correctional personnel, and other stakeholders in decision-making and negotiation of role responsibilities.

- Communicates consultation recommendations.

Standard 5D. Prescriptive Authority and Treatment

The advanced practice registered nurse uses prescriptive authority, procedures, referrals, treatments, and therapies in accordance with state and federal laws and regulations.

COMPETENCIES FOR THE ADVANCED PRACTICE REGISTERED NURSE

The advanced practice registered nurse:

- Prescribes evidence-based treatments, therapies, and procedures considering the patient's comprehensive healthcare needs.

- Prescribes pharmacological agents based on a current knowledge of pharmacology and physiology.

- Prescribes specific pharmacological agents and treatments based on clinical indicators, the patient's status and needs, and the results of diagnostic and laboratory tests.

- Evaluates therapeutic and potential adverse effects of pharmacological and nonpharmacological treatments.

- Provides patients with information about intended effects and potential adverse effects of proposed prescriptive therapies.

- Provides information about costs and alternative treatments and procedures, as appropriate.

- Evaluates and incorporates complementary and alternative therapies into education and practice.

Standard 6. Evaluation

The correctional registered nurse evaluates progress toward attainment of outcomes.

COMPETENCIES

The correctional registered nurse:

- Conducts a systematic, ongoing, and criterion-based evaluation of the outcomes in relation to the structures and processes prescribed by the plan and the indicated timeline.

- Collaborates in the evaluation process with the patient, family, other caregivers, and correctional staff who may be involved in the patient's living environment.

- Evaluates, in partnership with the patient, the effectiveness of the planned strategies in relation to the patient's responses and attainment of the expected outcomes.

- Uses ongoing assessment data to revise the diagnoses, outcomes, plan, and implementation as needed.

- Shares the results with the patient, other caregivers, and correctional staff who may be involved in the patient's living environment, in accordance with federal and state regulations.

- Participates in assessing and assuring responsible and appropriate use of interventions to minimize unwarranted or unwanted treatment and patient suffering.

- Documents the results of the evaluation.

ADDITIONAL COMPETENCIES FOR THE GRADUATE-LEVEL-PREPARED CORRECTIONAL NURSE AND THE APRN

The graduate-level-prepared correctional nurse or advanced practice registered nurse:

- Evaluates the accuracy of the diagnosis and the effectiveness of the interventions and other variables in relation to the patient's attainment of expected outcomes.

- Synthesizes the results of the evaluation to determine the effect of the plan on patients, families, groups, communities, and institutions.

- Adapts the plan of care and treatment according to the evaluation of patient response.

- Uses the results of the evaluation to make or recommend process and structural changes, including policy, procedure, and protocol revision, as appropriate.

Standards of Professional Performance for Correctional Nursing

Standard 7. Ethics

The correctional registered nurse practices ethically.

COMPETENCIES

The correctional registered nurse:

- Uses *Code of Ethics for Nurses with Interpretive Statements* (ANA, 2001) to guide practice.

- Delivers care in a manner that preserves and protects patient autonomy, dignity, rights, values, and beliefs.

- Recognizes the centrality of the patient and, when possible, the family, as core members of any healthcare team.

- Upholds patient confidentiality within legal and regulatory parameters.

- Assists patients in self-determination and informed decision-making.

- Maintains a therapeutic and professional nurse–patient relationship within appropriate professional role boundaries.

- Contributes to resolving ethical issues involving the patient, nurse colleagues, healthcare providers, correctional personnel, and other stakeholders.

- Takes appropriate action regarding instances of illegal, unethical, or inappropriate behavior that could endanger or jeopardize the best interests of the patient or situation.

- Speaks up when appropriate to question healthcare practice when necessary for safety and quality improvement.

- Advocates for equitable patient care.

ADDITIONAL COMPETENCIES FOR THE GRADUATE-LEVEL-PREPARED CORRECTIONAL NURSE AND THE APRN

The graduate-level-prepared correctional nurse or advanced practice registered nurse:

- Participates in interprofessional teams that address ethical risks, benefits, and outcomes.

- Provides information on the risks, benefits, and outcomes of healthcare regimens to allow informed decision-making by the patient, including informed consent and informed refusal.

Standard 8. Education

The correctional registered nurse attains knowledge and competence that reflect current nursing practice.

COMPETENCIES

The correctional registered nurse:

- Participates in ongoing educational activities related to appropriate knowledge bases and professional issues.

- Demonstrates a commitment to lifelong learning through self-reflection and inquiry to address learning and personal growth needs.

- Seeks experiences that reflect current practice to maintain knowledge, skills, abilities, and judgment in clinical practice or role performance.

- Acquires knowledge and skills appropriate to the role, population, specialty, setting, role, or situation.

- Seeks formal and independent learning experiences to develop and maintain clinical and professional skills and knowledge.

- Identifies learning needs based on nursing knowledge, the various roles the nurse may assume, and the changing needs of the population.

- Participates in formal or informal consultations to address issues in nursing practice as an application of education and knowledge base.

- Shares educational findings, experiences, and ideas with peers.

- Contributes to a work environment conducive to the education of healthcare professionals.

- Maintains professional records that provide evidence of competence and lifelong learning.

ADDITIONAL COMPETENCIES FOR THE GRADUATE-LEVEL-PREPARED CORRECTIONAL NURSE AND THE APRN

The graduate-level-prepared correctional nurse or advanced practice registered nurse:

- Uses current healthcare research findings and other evidence to promote and expand clinical knowledge, skills, abilities, and judgment; to enhance role performance; and to increase knowledge of professional issues.

Standard 9. Evidence-Based Practice and Research

The correctional registered nurse integrates evidence and research findings into practice.

COMPETENCIES

The correctional registered nurse:

- Utilizes current evidence-based nursing knowledge, including research findings, to guide practice.

- Incorporates evidence-based research when initiating changes in nursing practice.

- Participates, as appropriate to education level and position, in the formulation of evidence-based practice through research findings.

- Shares personal or third-party research findings with colleagues and peers.

ADDITIONAL COMPETENCIES FOR THE GRADUATE-LEVEL-PREPARED CORRECTIONAL NURSE AND THE APRN

The graduate-level-prepared correctional nurse or advanced practice registered nurse:

- Contributes to nursing knowledge by conducting or synthesizing research findings and other evidence that discovers, examines, and evaluates current practice, knowledge, theories, criteria, and creative approaches to improve healthcare outcomes.

- Promotes a climate of research and clinical inquiry.

- Disseminates research findings through activities such as presentations, publications, consultation, and journal clubs.

Standard 10. Quality of Practice

The correctional registered nurse contributes to quality nursing practice.

COMPETENCIES

The correctional registered nurse:

- Demonstrates quality by documenting the application of the nursing process in a responsible, accountable, and ethical manner.

- Uses creativity and innovation to enhance nursing care.

- Participates in quality improvement. Activities may include:

  - Identifying aspects of practice important for quality monitoring.

  - Using indicators to monitor quality, safety, and effectiveness of nursing practice.

  - Analyzing factors related to quality, safety, and effectiveness.

  - Collecting data to monitor quality and effectiveness of nursing practice.

  - Analyzing data to identify opportunities for improving nursing practice.

  - Formulating recommendations to improve nursing practice or outcomes.

  - Implementing activities to enhance the quality of nursing practice.

  - Developing policies, procedures, and guidelines to improve the quality of nursing practice.

  - Implementing policies, procedures, and guidelines to improve the quality of nursing practice.

  - Evaluating policies, procedures, and guidelines to improve the quality of nursing practice.

- Participating on interprofessional teams to evaluate clinical care or health services.

- Leading interprofessional teams to evaluate clinical care or health services.

- Participating in efforts to minimize costs and unnecessary duplication.

- Leading efforts to minimize costs and unnecessary duplication.

- Identifying problems that occur in work routines so as to correct process inefficiencies.*

- Analyzing organizational systems for barriers to quality patient outcomes.

- Implementing processes to remove or weaken barriers within organizational systems.

ADDITIONAL COMPETENCIES FOR THE GRADUATE-LEVEL-PREPARED CORRECTIONAL NURSE AND THE APRN

The graduate-level-prepared correctional nurse or advanced practice registered nurse:

- Provides leadership in the design and implementation of quality improvements.

- Designs innovations to effect positive change in practice and improve health outcomes.

- Evaluates the practice environment and quality of nursing care rendered in relation to existing evidence.

- Identifies opportunities for the generation and use of research and evidence.

- Obtains and maintains professional certification if it is available in the area of expertise.

- Uses the results of quality improvement to initiate changes in nursing practice and the healthcare delivery system.

* Board of Higher Education & Massachusetts Organization of Nurse Executives (BHE/MONE), 2006.

Standard 11. Communication

The correctional registered nurse communicates effectively in a variety of formats in all areas of practice.

COMPETENCIES

The correctional registered nurse:

- Assesses communication format preferences of the patient, families when possible, and colleagues.*

- Assesses her or his own communication skills in encounters with the patient, families, and colleagues.*

- Seeks continuous improvement of her or his own communication and conflict resolution skills.*

- Conveys information to the patient, families when possible, the inter-professional team, and others in communication formats that promote accuracy, understanding, confidentiality, and compliance with security regulations.

- Confirms the patient's understanding of the communication and message content.

- Questions the rationale supporting care processes and decisions when they do not appear to be in the best interest of the patient.*

- Discloses observations or concerns related to hazards and errors in care or the practice environment to the appropriate level.

- Maintains communication with other correctional professionals to minimize risks associated with transfers and transition in care delivery.

- Contributes her or his own professional perspective in discussions with the interprofessional team.

* BHE/MONE, 2006.

Standard 12. Leadership

The registered correctional nurse demonstrates leadership in the professional practice setting and the profession.

COMPETENCIES

The correctional registered nurse:

- Oversees the nursing care given by others while retaining accountability for the quality of care given to the patient.

- Abides by the vision, the associated goals, and the plan to implement and measure progress of an individual patient or progress within the context of the healthcare services rendered in the correctional organization.

- Demonstrates a commitment to continuous, lifelong learning, and education for self and others.

- Mentors colleagues for the advancement of nursing practice, the profession, and quality health care.

- Treats colleagues with respect, trust, and dignity.*

- Develops communication and conflict resolution skills.

- Participates in professional organizations.

- Communicates effectively with the patient and colleagues.

- Seeks ways to advance nursing autonomy and accountability.*

- Participates in efforts to influence healthcare policy involving patients and the profession.*

- Promotes the correctional nursing specialty within healthcare and correctional communities.

* BHE/MONE, 2006.

ADDITIONAL COMPETENCIES FOR THE GRADUATE-LEVEL-PREPARED CORRECTIONAL NURSE AND THE APRN

The graduate-level-prepared correctional nurse or advanced practice registered nurse:

- Influences decision-making bodies to improve the professional practice environment and patient outcomes.

- Provides direction to enhance the effectiveness of the interprofessional team.

- Promotes advanced practice nursing and role development by interpreting its role for patients, families, custody staff, and others.

- Models expert practice to interprofessional team members, patients, and custody staff.

- Mentors colleagues in the acquisition of clinical knowledge, skills, abilities, and judgment.

Standard 13. Collaboration

The correctional registered nurse collaborates with the patient, correctional facility administration, family, and other healthcare professionals in his or her conduct of nursing practice.

COMPETENCIES

The correctional registered nurse:

- Partners with other healthcare professionals, correctional facility administration and staff, family, and others to effect change and produce positive outcomes through the sharing of knowledge of the patient and/or situation.

- Communicates with the patient, correctional facility administration and staff, family, and other healthcare professionals regarding patient care and the role of the correctional registered nurse in that care.

- Promotes conflict management and engagement.

- Participates with other healthcare professionals, correctional facility administration and staff, family, and others in building consensus and/ or resolving conflict in the context of care of the patient.

- Applies group process and negotiation techniques with the patient, professional healthcare staff, family, and correctional facility administration and staff.

- Adheres to standards and applicable codes of conduct that govern behavior among peers and colleagues to create a work environment that promotes cooperation, respect, and trust.

- Cooperates with other healthcare professionals in creating a documented plan, focused on outcomes and decisions related to care and delivery of services, that indicates communication with the patient, family, correctional facility administration and staff, and others.

- Engages in teamwork and team-building processes.

ADDITIONAL COMPETENCIES FOR THE GRADUATE-LEVEL-PREPARED CORRECTIONAL NURSE AND THE APRN

The graduate-level-prepared correctional nurse or advanced practice registered nurse:

- Partners with others to enhance patient outcomes through interprofessional activities, such as education, consultation, management, technological development, or research opportunities.

- Invites the contribution of the patient, family, and team members in order to achieve optimal outcomes.

- Leads in establishing, improving, and sustaining collaborative relationships to achieve safe, quality patient care.

- Documents plan-of-care communications, rationales for plan-of-care changes, and collaborative discussions to improve patient outcomes.

Standard 14. Professional Practice Evaluation

The correctional registered nurse evaluates her or his own nursing practice in relation to professional practice standards and guidelines, relevant statutes, rules, and regulations.

COMPETENCIES

The correctional registered nurse:

- Provides age-appropriate and developmentally appropriate care in a culturally and ethnically sensitive manner.

- Engages in self-evaluation of practice on a regular basis by identifying areas of strength as well as areas in which professional growth would be beneficial.

- Obtains informal feedback regarding her or his own practice from patients, peers, professional colleagues, and others.

- Participates in peer review as appropriate.

- Takes action to achieve goals identified during the evaluation process.

- Provides evidence for practice decisions and actions as part of the informal and formal evaluation processes.

- Interacts with peers and colleagues to enhance her or his own professional nursing practice or role performance.

- Provides peers with formal or informal constructive feedback regarding their practice or role performance.

ADDITIONAL COMPETENCIES FOR THE GRADUATE-LEVEL-PREPARED CORRECTIONAL NURSE AND THE APRN

The graduate-level-prepared correctional nurse or advanced practice registered nurse:

- Engages in a formal process of seeking feedback regarding her or his own practice from patients, peers, professional colleagues, and others.

Standard 15. Resource Utilization

The correctional registered nurse utilizes appropriate resources to plan and provide nursing services that are safe, effective, and financially responsible.

COMPETENCIES

The correctional registered nurse:

- Assesses individual patient care needs and resources available to achieve desired outcomes.

- Identifies patient care needs, potential for harm, complexity of the task, and desired outcome when considering resource allocation.

- Delegates elements of care to appropriate healthcare workers in accordance with any applicable legal or policy parameters or principles.

- Identifies the evidence when evaluating resources.

- Advocates for resources, including technology, that enhance correctional nursing practice.

- Modifies practice when necessary to promote positive interaction among patients, care providers, correctional personnel, and technology.

- Assists the patient and, when possible, the family in identifying and securing appropriate services to address needs across the healthcare continuum.

- Assists the patient and, when possible, the family in factoring costs, risks, and benefits in decisions about treatment and care.

ADDITIONAL COMPETENCIES FOR THE GRADUATE-LEVEL-PREPARED CORRECTIONAL NURSE AND THE APRN

The graduate-level-prepared correctional nurse or advanced practice registered nurse:

- Utilizes organizational and community resources to formulate interprofessional plans of care.

- Formulates innovative solutions for patient care problems that utilize resources effectively and maintain quality.

- Designs evaluation strategies that demonstrate cost effectiveness, cost benefit, and efficiency factors associated with correctional nursing practice.

Standard 16. Environmental Health

The correctional registered nurse practices in an
environmentally safe and healthy manner.

"Environmental health addresses all the physical, chemical, and biological
factors external to a person, and all the related factors impacting behaviors.
It encompasses the assessment and control of those environmental factors
that can potentially affect health. It is targeted towards preventing disease
and creating health-supportive environments" [World Health Organization
(WHO), 2012].

COMPETENCIES

The correctional registered nurse:

- Attains knowledge of environmental health concepts, with implementation of environmental health strategies.

- Promotes a practice environment that reduces environmental health
risks for workers, patients, and others in the correctional setting.

- Assesses the practice environment for factors, such as sound, odor,
noise, and light, that may jeopardize health.

- Advocates for the judicious and appropriate use, storage, and disposal of
products in health care.

- Communicates environmental health risks and exposure reduction
strategies to patients, families, colleagues, and communities.

- Utilizes scientific evidence to determine if a product or treatment is an
environmental risk.

- Participates in strategies to promote healthy communities.

ADDITIONAL COMPETENCIES FOR THE GRADUATE-LEVEL-PREPARED CORRECTIONAL NURSE AND THE APRN

The graduate-level-prepared correctional nurse or advanced practice registered nurse:

- Creates partnerships that promote sustainable environmental health policies and conditions.

- Analyzes the impact of social, political, and economic influences on the environment and human health exposures.

- Critically evaluates the manner in which environmental health issues are presented by the popular media.

- Advocates for implementation of environmental principles for nursing practice.

- Supports nurses in advocating for and implementing environmental principles for nursing practice

References and Bibliography

American Academy of Pediatrics. (2011, December). Policy statement: Health care for youth in the juvenile justice system. *Pediatrics, 128*(6), 1219–1235.

American Corrections Association (ACA). (2002). Declaration of principles. Retrieved May 3, 2012, from http://www.aca.org/adaview.asp?pageid=447

American Nurses Association (ANA). (2001). *Code of Ethics for Nurses with interpretive statements.* Silver Spring, MD: Nursesbooks.org.

American Nurses Association (ANA). (2010). *Nursing: Scope and standards of practice* (2nd ed.). Silver Spring, MD: Nursesbooks.org.

Anno, B. J. (1997). Health behaviors in prisons and correctional facilities. In David S. Gochman (Ed.), *Handbook of health behaviors research, Vol. III: Demography, development, and diversity,* Ch. 14. New York, NY: Plenum Press.

Anno, B. J. (2001). *Correctional health care guidelines for the management of an adequate delivery system.* Washington, DC: National Institute of Corrections, U.S. Department of Justice.

Baral Abrams, G., Etkind, P., Burke, M. C., & Cram, V. (2008, April). Sexual violence and subsequent risk of sexually transmitted disease among incarcerated women. *Journal of Correctional Health Care, 14*(2), 80–88.

Binswanger, I. A., Krueger, P. M., & Steiner, J. F. (2009). Prevalence of chronic medical conditions among jail and prison inmates in the USA compared with the general population. *Journal of Epidemiology & Community Health, 63,* 912–919.

Blair, P. (2000). Improving nursing practice in correctional settings. *Journal of Nursing Law, 7*(2), 19–30.

Board of Higher Education & Massachusetts Organization of Nurse Executives (BHE/MONE). (2006, March 23–24). *Creativity and connections: Building the framework for the future of nursing education.* Report from the Invitational Working Session, Burlington, MA: MONE. Retrieved from http://www.mass.edu/currentinit/documents /NursingCreativityAndConnections.pdf

Bureau of Justice Statistics (BJS). (2011, December 15). Total correctional population—US correctional population declined for second consecutive year. Retrieved from http://www.bjs.gov

Burrow, G., Knox, C., & Villanueva, H. (2006). Nursing in the primary care setting. In M. Puisis, *Clinical practice in correctional medicine* (2nd ed.) (pp. 426–459). Philadelphia, PA: Mosby Elsevier.

Cardwell, A., & Gilmore, M. (2011). County jails and the Affordable Health Care Act: Enrolling eligible individuals in health coverage. Retrieved from http://www.naco.org/programs/csd/Documents/Health%20Reform%20 Implementation/County-Jails-HealthCare_WebVersion.pdf

Centers for Disease Control and Prevention (CDC). (2003, October 17). Methicillin-resistant Staphylococcus aureus infections in correctional facilities—Georgia, California, and Texas, 2001–2003. *MMWR, (55)*RR09, 992–996.

Centers for Disease Control and Prevention (CDC). (2006, July 7). Prevention and control of tuberculosis in correctional and detention facilities: Recommendations from CDC, *MMWR, (55)*RR09, 1–44. Retrieved from http://www.cdc.gov/mmwr/preview/mmwrhtml/rr5509a1.htm

Centers for Disease Control and Prevention (CDC). (2011, May 20). Surveillance of health status in minority communities: Racial and ethnic approaches to community health across the U.S. (REACH US) Risk Factor Survey, United States 2009. *MMWR Recommendations & Reports, 60*(SS06), 1–41.

Centers for Disease Control and Prevention (CDC). (2012). Correctional facilities & viral hepatitis. Retrieved from http://www.cdc.gov/hepatitis /Settings/Corrections.htm

Gibbons, J. J., & Katzenbach, J. T. (2006, June). *Confronting confinement: A report of the Commission on Safety and Abuse in America's Prisons.*

New York, NY: Vera Institute of Justice. Retrieved from http://www.vera.org /pubs/confronting-confinement

Goldkuhle, U. (1999). Health service utilization by women in prison: Health needs indicators and response effects. *Journal of Correctional Health Care, 1*, 63–83.

Haigler, K., Harlowe, C., O'Connor, P., & Campbell, A. (1994, October). *Literacy behind prison walls: Profiles of the prison population from the National Adult Literacy Survey* (Office of Educational Research and Improvement, NCES 1994-102). Washington, DC: U.S. Department of Education. Retrieved from http://nces.ed.gov/pubs94/94102.pdf

Hammett, T. (2006, June). HIV/AIDS and other infectious diseases among correctional inmates: Transmission, burden and an appropriate response. *American Journal of Public Health, 96*(6), 974–978.

Hayes, L. M. (2009, February). *Juvenile suicide in confinement: A national survey.* (OJJDP Report). National Center on Institutions and Alternatives NCJ213691 Stats paragraph 1. Retrieved from http://www/ncjrs.gov/App /Publications/abstract.aspx?ID=234394

HCV Advocate. (2003).Hepatitis C infection in prisons. (William Cassidy, M.D.; Louisiana State University Health Science Center.) Retrieved from www.hcvadvocate.org/hcsp/articles/cassidy-1.html

Health Resources and Services Administration (HRSA), U.S. Department of Health and Human Services. (2000). *The registered nurse population. March 2000 findings from the National Sample Survey of Registered Nurses.* Retrieved from http://bhpr.hrsa.gov/healthworkforce/rnsurveys /rnsurvey2000.pdf

Health Resources and Services Administration (HRSA), U.S. Department of Health and Human Services. (2004). *The registered nurse population: Findings from the March 2004 National Sample Survey of Registered Nurses.* Retrieved from http://bhpr.hrsa.gov/healthworkforce/rnsurveys /rnsurvey2004.pdf

Health Resources and Services Administration (HRSA), U.S. Department of Health and Human Services. (2010, September). *The registered nurse population: Findings from the 2008 National Sample Survey of Registered Nurses.* Retrieved from http://bhpr.hrsa.gov/healthworkforce/ rnsurveys/rnsurveyfinal.pdf

Institute of Medicine (IOM). (2011). *The future of nursing: Leading change, advancing health.* Washington, DC: National Academies Press. Retrieved from http://www.iom.edu/Reports/2010/The-Future-of-Nursing -Leading-Change-Advancing-Health.aspx

Kesler, J. (2012). Telemedicine: A viable solution. *Correctional Health Report, 13*(3), 33–48.

Knight, D. (2009). Electronic medical records moving jails forward. *Correctional Health Report, 10*(4), 49–64.

Kokontis, M. (2007). Dorothea Dix, student, reformer, and crusader: Constructing the past. *Digital Commons, 8*(1), article 5. Retrieved from http://digitalcommons.iwu.edu/constructing/vol8/iss1/5

Krohn, L. T., Corrigan, J. M., & Donaldson, M. S. (Eds.). (2000). *To err is human: Building a safer system.* Retrieved from http://books.nap.edu /catalog/9728.html

LaMarre, M. (2006). Nursing role and practice in correctional facilities. In M. Puisis, *Clinical practice in correctional medicine* (2nd ed.) (pp. 417–424). Philadelphia, PA: Mosby Elsevier.

Lasko, M. (2012). Multiculturalism in a correctional environment. *Correctional Health Report, 13*(40), 49–64.

Loeb, S. J., & AbuDagga, A. (2006). Health related research on older inmates: An integrative review. *Research in Nursing & Health, 29,* 556–565.

Malcolm, B. (2011, July). The rise of methicillin-resistant Staphylococcus aureus in U.S. correctional populations. *Journal of Correctional Health Care, 17*(3), 254–263.

Mauer, M., & King, R. (2007, July). *Uneven justice: State rates of incarceration by race and ethnicity.* Washington, DC: The Sentencing Project. Retrieved from http://advancabag.com/documents /rd_stateratesofincbyraceandethnicity.pdf

Murtha, R. (1975). Change in one city's system: It started with a director of nursing. *American Journal of Nursing, 75*(3), 421–422.

Muse, M. (2009). Correctional nursing: The evolution of a specialty. *Correctional Care, 23*(1), 3–4.

National Commission on Correctional Health Care (NCCHC). (2002). *The health status of soon-to-be-released inmates: A report to Congress*, Vol. I. Chicago, IL: Author. Retrieved from http://www.ncchc.org/pubs /pubs_stbr.vol1.html

National Commission on Correctional Health Care (NCCHC). (2008a). *Standards for health services in jails*. Chicago, IL: Author.

National Commission on Correctional Health Care (NCCHC). (2008b). *Standards for health services in prisons*. Chicago, IL: Author.

Office of Juvenile Justice and Delinquency Programs (OJJDP). (2011). Juvenile arrests 2009. Juvenile Offenders and Victims National Report Series Bulletin NCJ 236477.

Pew Center on the States. (2008, February). *One in 100: Behind bars in America 2008* (Public Safety Performance Project, Pew Charitable Trust) (pp. 1–35).Retrieved from http://www.pewcenteronthestates.org /uploadedFiles/8015PCTS_Prison08_FINAL_2-1-1_FORWEB.pdf

Pinta, E. (2011). Prevalence rates for mental disorders in prisons: Implications and treatment programs. *Correctional Health Report, 12*(4), 49–64.

Posner, M. (1992). The *Estelle* medical profession judgment standard: The right of those in state custody to receive high-cost medical treatments. *American Journal of Law & Medicine, 18*(4), 347–368.

Prison terminal: Life and death in a prison hospice. (n.d.). The aging prison population. Retrieved from http://www.prisonterminal.com/essays%20 aging%20prison%20pop.html

Reddi, V. (2005). *Dorothea Lynde Dix (1802–1887)*. Retrieved from http://www.nursingadvocacy.org/press/pioneers/dix.html

Reimer, G. (2008, July). The graying of the U.S. prisoner population. *Journal of Correctional Health Care, 14*(3), 202–208.

Rich, J., Wohl, D., Beckwith, C., Spaulding, A., Lepp, N., Baillargeon, J., Gardner, A., Avery, A., Altice, F., & Springer, S. (2011, December). HIV-related research in correctional populations: Now is the time. *Current HIV/AIDS Report, 8*(4), 288–296.

Schoenly, L. (2011). Legal history of correctional nursing. *Correctional Health*. Retrieved from http://www.nursinglink.monster.com/education /articles/1401-legal-history-of-correction-nursing

Shelton, D. (2009). Forensic nursing in secure environments. *Journal of Forensic Nursing, 5*, 131–142.

Shelton, D., Weiskopf, C., & Nicholson, M. (2010). Correctional nursing competency development in the Connecticut correctional managed health care program. *Journal of Correctional Health Care, 16*(4), 38–47.

Sloan, C. D., & Johnson, J. D. (2012). Legal origin and issues behind correctional nursing. Retrieved from http://www.ce.nurse.com /RetailCourseView.aspx

Smyer, T., & Burbank, P. M. (2009, December). The U.S. correctional system and the older prisoner. *Journal of Gerontological Nursing, 35*(12), 32–37.

Spaulding, A., Seals, R., Page, M., Brzozowski, A. K., Rhodes, W., & Hammett, T. (2009, November).PLoS ONE, *4*(11), e7558, pp. 1–8. Retrieved from www.plosone.org

Torrey, E. F., Kennard, A. D., Eslinger, D., Lamb, R., & Pavle, J. (2010, May). *More mentally ill persons are in jails and prisons than hospitals: A survey of the states.* Arlington, VA: Treatment Advocacy Center. Retrieved from http://www.treatmentadvocacycenter.org/storage/documents /final_jails_v_hospitals_study.pdf

Weiskopf, C. (2005). Nurses' experience of caring for inmate patients. *Journal of Advanced Nursing, 49*(4), 336–343.

Wilper, A. P., Woolhandler, S., Wesley Boyd, J., Lasser, K. E., McCormick, D., Bor, D. H., & Himmelstein, D. U. (2009). The health and health care of US prisoners: Results of a nationwide survey. *American Journal of Public Health, 99*(4), 666–672.

Women's Prison Association (WPA). (2009). *Institute on Women and Criminal and Justice, Quick Facts: Women and criminal justice, 2009.* Retrieved from http://wpaonline.org/pdf/Quick%20Facts%20 Women%20and%20CJ%202009.pdf

World Health Organization (WHO). (2012). Environmental health. Retrieved from http://www.who.int/topics/environmental_health/en/

Appendix A.

Corrections Nursing: Scope and Standards of Practice (2007)

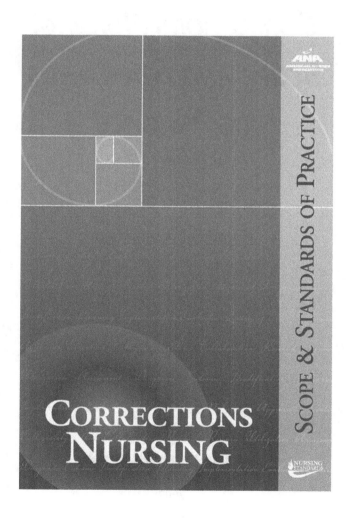

The content in this appendix is not current and is of historical significance only.

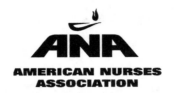

**AMERICAN NURSES
ASSOCIATION**

CORRECTIONS NURSING:
SCOPE AND STANDARDS
OF PRACTICE

The Publishing Program of ANA

AMERICAN NURSES ASSOCIATION
SILVER SPRING, MARYLAND
2007

The content in this appendix is not current and is of historical significance only.

ACKNOWLEDGMENTS

Work Group Members

Kleanthe Caruso, MSN, RN, CCHP, CNAA, BC, Chairperson
Kathleen Bachmeier, MS, RN, BC
Patricia Blair, JD, LLM, MSN, RN
Arlene Chapman, RN, CCHP
Margaret M. Collatt, BSN, RN, CCHP-A
Catherine I. Fogel, PhD, RN,C, WHNCNP
Gail W. Fricks, BA, RN, CCHP
Rob Hofacre, BSN, MCRP, RN
JoRene Kerns, BSN, RN, CCHP
Jane McNeely, ARNP
Jacqueline Moore, PhD, RN, CCHP-A
Sue Moul, RN, CCHP-A
Mary Muse, MSN, RN, CCHP
M. Kay Northrup, BSN, RN, CCHP
Barbara Skeen, RN

ANA Staff

Carol J. Bickford, PhD, RN,BC—Content editor
Yvonne Daley Humes, MSA—Project coordinator
Matthew Seiler, RN, Esq.—Legal counsel

Winifred Carson-Smith, JD—Consultant

The content in this appendix is not current and is of historical significance only.

CONTENTS

The content in this appendix is not current and is of historical significance only.

The content in this appendix is not current and is of historical significance only.

PREFACE

In 2002 the American Nurses Association convened the volunteer work group of registered nurses tasked with the responsibility to review and revise the 1995 *Scope and Standards of Nursing Practice in Correctional Facilities*. The nurses held various positions in state and local adult and juvenile corrections and detention facilities, academic institutions, professional organizations, and healthcare facilities, and contributed a diverse perspective in all discussions.

The work group used *Code of Ethics for Nurses with Interpretive Statements* (2001); *Nursing's Social Policy Statement, 2nd Edition* (2003); and *Nursing: Scope and Standards of Practice* (2004) as foundational resources and completed its work via telephone conference calls and electronic mail communications. In 2004 a draft document was posted at ANA's web site (www.NursingWorld.org) for a 60-day public comment period. The work group reviewed each resultant comment and further revised the draft as necessary. In 2006 the Congress on Nursing Practice Committee on Nursing Practice Standards and Guidelines completed two reviews of the draft *Corrections Nursing: Scope and Standards of Practice* against established review criteria. Recommended revisions were completed before the ANA's Congress on Nursing Practice and Economics conducted a final review in fall 2006. The edits recommended by the Congress members to improve clarity have also been incorporated.

The content in this appendix is not current and is of historical significance only.

Corrections Nursing: Scope of Practice

Corrections nursing is the practice of nursing and the delivery of patient care within the unique and distinct environment of the criminal justice system. The criminal justice system includes jails, prisons, juvenile detention centers, substance abuse treatment facilities, and other facilities.

Health Care in Correctional System Settings

Through most of its history, the United States corrections system had little or no health care available to inmates, as the courts typically took a detached approach to correctional issues and avoided interfering in the administration and operation of correctional facilities. This gave corrections administrators enormous freedom with little regulation or accountability imposed on daily operations. Public interest was minimal, and government agencies saw no reason to pour tax money into the prison system. The lack of oversight contributed to serious abuses behind the walls of correctional institutions.

The civil rights movement in the 1960s focused public attention on reform and improving conditions for the less fortunate. The inevitable scrutiny of conditions and practices in correctional facilities forced the American judicial system to begin to respond to inmate claims.

In 1976, the United States Supreme Court established a constitutional standard for inmate health care in the Texas case, *Estelle v. Gamble*. Inmate Gamble claimed that prison officials inflicted undue suffering on him when they failed to provide adequate care for an injury sustained in prison. The court ruled that "... deliberate indifference to serious medical needs of prisoners constitutes the 'unnecessary and wanton infliction of pain,' *Gregg v. Georgia, supra,* at 173 (joint opinion), proscribed by the Eighth Amendment. This is true whether the indifference is manifested by prison doctors in their response to the prisoner's needs or by prison guards in intentionally denying or delaying access to medical care or intentionally interfering with the treatment once prescribed. Regardless of how evidenced, deliberate indifference to a prisoner's serious illness or injury states a cause of action under § 1983" (*Estelle v. Gamble* 1976).

The decision led to several reforms in inmate litigation that included the following list of inmate rights related to health care:

- The right to access care
- The right to professional judgment
- The right to care that is ordered
- The right to informed consent
- The right to refuse treatment
- The right to medical confidentiality

Federal enforcement of these rights forced correctional agencies to re-structure their inmate healthcare systems. During the years since *Estelle v. Gamble*, the development of both case law and national standards on correctional health care have affirmed that prisoners had a right to be free of "deliberate indifference to their serious healthcare needs."

Population Served

At the end of 2005, over 7 million people were on probation, in jail or prison, or on parole. This represents 3.2% of all U.S. adult residents or one out of every 32 adults. After dramatic increases in the 1980s and 1990s, the incarceration rate has leveled off at an average annual increase of 3.4% (Bureau of Justice Statistics 2004). The June 2004 Juvenile Offenders and Victims National Report Series indicated that an esti-mated 134,011 youth were held in 2,939 facilities on October 27, 1999 (U.S. Department of Justice 2004). That total does not include juveniles under the age of 18 who are held in adult facilities.

Today's inmates are older and sicker and remain imprisoned longer when compared to the inmates of 20 years ago. In general, inmates come from socioeconomic groups at high risk for poor health and have not had access to regular healthcare services or proper treatment for medical conditions. They also have a disproportionately greater num-ber of chronic illnesses and infectious diseases than the non-incarcer-ated population.

The incidence of HIV/AIDS in prisons and jails is substantially higher than in the population at large due to an over-representation of those with a history of high-risk behaviors. The CDC reports that in 1997 approximately 17% of all persons with the human immunodeficiency virus (HIV) had been released from corrections facilities (www.cdc.gov). As of 2001, state and federal prisoners known to be positive for HIV and confirmed AIDS cases totaled 24,147 (21,268 male and 2,265 female) (*Sourcebook of Criminal Justice Statistics* 2003).

Tuberculosis is one of the most threatening infectious diseases facing correctional systems. An estimated 35% of all persons with active TB cases in 1996 passed through the correctional system. In 2002 the National Commission on Correctional Health Care reported that the prevalence of active TB among inmates is between 4 and 17 times greater than among the total U.S. population (NCCHC 2002, p. xi). A study of U.S. surveillance data from 1993 to 2003 showed that 3.7% of all TB cases were reported within correctional systems. TB case rates for federal and state prisons were 29.4% and 24.3% per 100,000, respectively, compared to 6.7% per 100,000 in the general population. Inmates with TB also are more likely than the general population to forgo treatment (MacNeil 2005).

Hepatitis C, identified in 1989, has infected an estimated 3.9 million Americans. The most common form of transmission is through intravenous drug use. Approximately 83% of the nation's drug users are incarcerated at some time, and research indicates that 80% of inmates have a history of substance abuse (NCCHC 2002).

Advances in health care, longer prison terms, mandatory sentences, and more restrictive policies are keeping inmates in prison longer with lower chances of parole. This results in a much older resident population. "From 1992 to January 1, 2001, the number of state and federal inmates age 50 and older increased from 41,586 to 113,358, a staggering increase of 172.6%" (Anno et al. 2004, p. 7). In 2004 almost 240,000 inmates in our nation's prisons were age 45–54 and more than 16,000 were age 55 or older (American Correctional Association 2005a). In 2005, the average proportion of elderly inmates in state prison systems was 5.36% (American Correctional Association 2005b).

Inmates suffer from age-related conditions earlier in life. Personal histories of poor nutrition, lack of preventive care, and high-risk behavior such as smoking and drug use are all common in the general incarcerated population. This makes a 50-year-old inmate's health status comparable to that of a 65-year-old living in the community.

The content in this appendix is not current and is of historical significance only.

Women are the fastest growing segment of the correctional population. At year end 2003, the 101,179 women in prison comprised 6.9% of the state and federal prison population (Bureau of Justice Statistics 2004). Although more than half of these women are under the age of 35, the majority have unhealthy past lifestyles which include drug and alcohol abuse, sex work, and multiple partners, which put them at high risk for chronic and communicable diseases (Anno 1997).

In addition to basic healthcare needs, these women have special healthcare needs associated with their reproductive systems and thus pose a great challenge in the correctional healthcare system geared to house male inmates. Approximately 6% are pregnant on admission to jails and prisons and account for an estimated 8,820 of the 3.8 million births in the United States each year. Due to unhealthy lifestyles prior to incarceration, most of these pregnancies are classified as high risk (Greenfeld and Snell 1999). In a 2003 survey, pelvic exams, prenatal/postpartum services, mammograms, and pap smears were provided in all state systems surveyed, while reproductive counseling was offered in 77% of the reporting systems (American Correctional Association 2004).

Gender differences continue, with women having higher rates of diabetes, HIV, and sexually transmitted diseases, as well as higher rates of serious mental illnesses, drug abuse, depression, and other emotional problems in comparison with the male population. Consequently this results in women offenders using healthcare services more frequently than do their male counterparts (Goldkuhle 1999).

The deinstitutionalization of persons with mental illness over the last several decades has had a dramatic impact on the corrections environment. New therapies, decreased insurance reimbursements, and tightening state and local healthcare budgets have resulted in decreased length of stay and a drastic reduction in the number of state and county mental hospitals and inpatient beds. In 1970, there were approximately 368,000 beds in mental institutions. By 1992 that number had decreased to 84,000 beds. Lack of available community financial and social system supports has therefore resulted in persons with mental illness often becoming nomads who eventually end up residing in ever-increasing numbers in America's jails and prisons. Estimates indicate that 10–20% of inmate populations are suffering from major psychiatric disorders and require mental health services.

The content in this appendix is not current and is of historical significance only.

Nurses in the Corrections Environment

The history of corrections nursing began as early as 1797 with the opening of the New York City Newgate Prison. Its warden, Thomas Eddy, believed that criminals could be rehabilitated, and he established a school for the inmates as well as the first prison hospital and pharmacy. However, nursing as a professional presence in the correctional setting did not appear until the 1960s, and it began to gain visibility toward the end of the twentieth century.

Rena Murtha, a pioneer in corrections nursing, described entering a large correctional facility where the nurse was perceived as a "tool of the warden, a slave of the physician and an unknown to the patient" (1975). Since that time, corrections nursing practice has evolved into a variety of essential roles ranging from primary health care to management and administration. Today's corrections nurse is a respected member of the correctional system staff.

Just as it is difficult to ascertain the numbers and characteristics of the corrections population, this nursing specialty continues to be hidden in the statistical reporting about nurses and their employment and work settings. For example, the only reference to this nursing specialty in the 2000 National Sample Survey of Registered Nurses is the projected number of 18,033 registered nurses working in prisons or jails (USDHHS 2002). The *Sourcebook of Criminal Justice Statistics 2003* does not report the numbers of registered nurses or other healthcare providers working in correctional settings in its statistics and tables. Likewise, the American public is unaware of the complex conditions and great strains that face nurses working in correctional healthcare settings.

Correctional systems are under increasing pressure from the courts to provide adequate and humane levels of health care with limited resources and little public sympathy. Social and political conditions facing nurses in these settings are demanding and appeal to the noblest of humanitarian instincts. Nurses are often the foundation of the correctional healthcare system and in many cases the only providers of healthcare services in those systems. Correctional systems meet their responsibility to provide adequate and safe healthcare services to those incarcerated by using the expertise and unique knowledge and skills of registered nurses.

The content in this appendix is not current and is of historical significance only.

Nurses can often experience personal and professional conflict in these practice settings. In many cases, nurses are direct employees of the correctional facility and may be in the same organizational hierarchy as the correctional officers. On one hand, they are employees of an institution whose mission is security and public safety. On the other hand, they are healthcare providers whose mission is health and wellness. There is firm support in national standards to support the restriction of nurse participation in activities related strictly to security (NCCHC 2002). The focus on security may, at times, conflict with the provision of health services. For example, the goals of security may create a condition of conflict by considering healthcare access to be a privilege versus a right.

The registered nurse is an essential part of the correctional system and faces the daily challenges of providing health care in that setting. It is imperative that nurses in correctional settings recognize their professional responsibility for role development and clarification based on a commitment to quality nursing care according to recognized standards. The American Nurses Association and other organizations, such as the American Correctional Health Services Association, the American Correctional Association, and the Academy of Correctional Health Professionals, are membership organizations that serve as a forum for current issues and needs confronting corrections nurses. As the correctional system grows and continues to evolve, the corrections nurse will remain the advocate to ensure that patients are at an optimal state of physical and mental health to become productive citizens when they rejoin the community.

Principles of Corrections Nursing

Nursing is the protection, promotion, and optimization of health and abilities, prevention of illness and injury, alleviation of suffering through the diagnosis and treatment of human response, and advocacy in the care of individuals, families, communities, and populations (ANA 2004, p. 7). Nursing is a science and an art, the essence of which is caring for and respecting human beings, including those in the corrections environment. The following principles serve as the underpinning for corrections nursing:

- A registered nurse's primary duty in the corrections setting is to restore and maintain the health of patients in a spirit of compassion, concern, and professionalism.

The content in this appendix is not current and is of historical significance only.

- Each patient, regardless of circumstances, possesses intrinsic value and should be treated with dignity and respect.

- Each encounter with patients and families should portray professionalism, compassion, and concern.

- Each patient should receive quality care that is cost-effective and consistent with the latest treatment parameters and clinical guidelines.

- Patient confidentiality and privacy should be preserved.

- Nurses should collaborate with other healthcare team members, correctional staff, and community colleagues to meet the holistic needs of patients, which include physical, psychosocial, and spiritual aspects of care.

- Nurses should encourage each individual through patient and family education to take responsibility for disease prevention and health promotion.

- Each nurse maintains responsibility for monitoring and evaluating nursing practice necessary for continuous quality improvement.

- Nursing leadership should promote the highest quality of patient care through application of fair and equitable policies and procedures in collaboration with other healthcare services team members and corrections staff.

- Nursing services should be guided by nurse administrators who foster professional and personal development. These responsible leaders are sensitive to employee needs; give support, praise, and recognition; and encourage continuing education, participation in professional organizations, and generation of knowledge through research.

Role of the Corrections Nurse

Registered nurses working in corrections settings must demonstrate the essence of nursing in a practice setting and work environment that does not have health care as its primary mission. The care and judgment required to meet patients' needs rest with the nurse's assessment. Matters of nursing judgment are solely the domain of the registered nurse and may be challenged in such an environment without a supporting healthcare services infrastructure.

The incarcerated vary from youth to aged adults, include men and women, and are individuals of all racial and ethnic backgrounds who are often disenfranchised, economically challenged, educationally limited, and largely ignored by society. These people frequently enter the corrections system with communicable and chronic diseases and complications resulting from a previous lack of appropriate healthcare services. Corrections nurses work to limit the healthcare disparities experienced by this unique and extremely diversified corrections population.

Corrections nurses are expected to deliver care to all patients with compassion, empathy, commitment, competency, dedication, and a positive attitude. Although the length of incarceration differs in the various settings, corrections nurses play an integral role in providing healthcare services to this population through patient education, patient advocacy, and the delivery of patient care.

It is inappropriate for nurses to be involved in the security aspects of the facility and disciplinary decisions or committees. Corrections nurses must be vigilant in maintaining a healthcare role and not participate in nontherapeutic court-ordered procedures, such as but not limited to body cavity searches or executions by lethal injections, performed solely for correctional purposes and without informed consent.

Nursing Practice in Correctional Settings

Correctional health care is one of the fastest growing specialties in health services today and offers new and unique roles for nursing in the evolving correctional healthcare settings. Because healthcare services are offered within community corrections facilities, jails, juvenile detention centers, and both juvenile and adult correctional institutions, the registered nurse must be prepared to address a wide spectrum of needs, including those associated with women's health, the pediatric through geriatric age continuum, and end-of-life care of patients in corrections settings. Such corrections facilities can house fewer than 50 juveniles or adults, or thousands of adult inmates. The majority of large adult correctional systems have one or more specialized facilities.

Most detainees do not need frequent or ongoing nursing care, and the registered nurse is not usually involved in assisting with activities of daily living except for those services required in infirmaries, skilled nursing or extended care areas or facilities, and hospital settings. Almost

The content in this appendix is not current and is of historical significance only.

all adult incarcerated offenders need at least occasional nursing services for the treatment of injuries, flu symptoms, back pain, headache, etc. Many also need nursing evaluations subsequent to altercations with other inmates, use of force, segregation placement, mental health crises, and/or other such intermittent circumstances.

Nurses usually interact with inmates in clinic areas or inmate housing units, but they may need to provide emergency care for patients in both indoor and outdoor work sites, recreational facilities, classrooms, dining facilities, visiting rooms, and other common areas. Real-life examples of such emergent care instances reported by experienced corrections nurses include delivery of a baby in the women's shower, farm injuries (one inmate was gored by a boar, another was trampled by a steer, and another fell off a barn roof), and industrial injuries (one inmate got his fingers caught in a router, one cut off the tips of his fingers with a saw, another caught his hand in an ironing press, and another got metal splinters in his eye while working in a metal shop).

The major emphasis of nursing care in most correctional settings is the provision of primary care services for the juvenile or adult population. These services are comparable to the care and surveillance services requiring the skills characteristic of public health, community health, occupational health, ambulatory care, emergency, and school nurses. Clinical settings include outpatient and urgent care clinics, acute care, skilled nursing, and long-term care inpatient healthcare facilities. Primary health services include the provision of intake evaluations, health screenings, direct healthcare services, analyzing individual health behaviors, teaching, counseling, and assisting individuals in assuming responsibility for their own health to the best of their ability, knowledge, and circumstances. Specialized mental health and chemical dependency units and facilities, critical care, neurological trauma, and dialysis services may supplement the primary care resources and require appropriately prepared specialty registered nurses and advanced practice registered nurses.

Registered nurses, as the primary healthcare providers in correctional settings, are challenged to provide health education and health promotion activities, evaluate the effectiveness of planned care, encourage preventive behavior, and address other public health issues within the prison setting. In addition, the registered nurse coordinates the linkage to community heathcare resources prior to the offender's release from incarceration, a critical function that provides the inmate the opportunity for continuity of care and helps facilitate a successful return to the community.

General Nursing Practice

The needs of the correctional population demand that the corrections nurse have a sound background preparation in community/public health, psychiatric, emergency, disease management and chronic care, medical-surgical and, in some settings, critical care nursing. Skills in negotiation, problem solving, listening, and communication are invaluable.

The registered nurse in corrections must be able to demonstrate good assessment and organizational skills as well as critical decision-making and thinking skills, especially when serving in the role of the only healthcare provider on site. Facility protocols and provider-generated order sets provide direction for the healthcare activities and specific patient care measures. However, such structures do not allow the corrections nurse to abdicate one's professional nursing responsibility for appropriate assessment, critical thinking, decision-making, and patient advocacy activities.

The registered nurse, in addition to providing direct nursing care, assesses the patient's health status, analyzes the assessment data, develops or modifies diagnoses, develops or modifies the plan of care based on those assessments and diagnoses, and evaluates the effectiveness of the plan of care. The corrections nurse often cares for patients with multiple and complex health conditions and diagnoses requiring an increased intensity of healthcare resources. The necessary associated nursing activities include patient assessment; decisions about medication, treatment delivery, and assessment of their effects; crisis intervention; triage; education; and patient advocacy. Scheduling of appointments, transportation, and other resources may require complex planning and the negotiation of staff and fiscal resources.

Nursing care within the corrections setting may be provided in collaboration with other nurses and health professionals, or independently, which is most often the case in a small or rural facility. Nursing care may be provided by a team of nurses with differing levels of preparation and licensure, including the registered nurse, advanced practice registered nurse, and licensed practical nurse. The preferred educational preparation of the registered nurse for entry into corrections nursing practice

The content in this appendix is not current and is of historical significance only.

is at the baccalaureate level. Continuing professional development is expected, including further educational preparation to achieve a baccalaureate or graduate-level degree.

Correctional facilities vary in size and configuration. The overriding mission of security, with its locks, cameras, bars, correctional officers, and searches creates an environment of noise, distractions, and confusion which must be appropriately managed to maintain a therapeutic environment for nursing care. For example, consider how medication administration by nurses differs in this non-healthcare environment. In corrections settings medication administration may be accomplished by what is referred to in some settings as a "pill line" where the patient comes to the medication area and receives the necessary therapy. Large numbers of patients and large numbers of medications or treatments may require that nurses negotiate care delivery and medication administration times and may also increase the potential for errors that result with interruptions and distractions. Such patient encounters may necessitate unscheduled time allocations for reassessment and educational intervention opportunities.

Nursing practice must be balanced with the goals of corrections and the incarcerated person's rights to appropriate health care. If the patient cannot present for healthcare services because of disability, injury, or seclusion restrictions, the corrections nurse must go to the patient's location, conduct an appropriate and timely assessment, render or secure appropriate healthcare services, and accurately complete the necessary documentation record(s). The published *Standards for Health Services in Correctional Institutions* of the American Public Health Association (APHA 2003), the American Correctional Association and the National Commission on Correctional Health Care standards, along with state laws and state nurse practice acts and regulations, can provide guidance and support for the corrections nurse.

Working inside a correctional setting requires that the corrections nurse have knowledge of the legal aspects of nursing and litigation related to correctional health care. The corrections nurse must be acutely aware of the need for appropriate documentation of care rendered. Maintaining confidentiality of patient health information often requires special attention, especially when corrections staff must assist in monitoring the health status of patients.

The content in this appendix is not current and is of historical significance only.

The corrections nurse is expected to demonstrate integrity and highly ethical and moral practice, appreciating the legally mandated obligation to deliver nursing care regardless of the individual's circumstances or offenses. The basic concept of patient advocacy may be foreign to the corrections environment and may need to be regularly reaffirmed by the corrections nurse.

The licensed practical or vocational nurse, in accordance with the licensure laws of the state and under the direction of a registered nurse or advanced practice clinician, provides basic nursing care, collaborates with other members of the healthcare team in the development and implementation of a nursing plan of care, and contributes to an evaluation of the effectiveness of that plan.

Advanced Practice Registered Nurse

The advanced practice registered nurse (APRN) roles include the clinical nurse specialist (CNS), nurse practitioner (NP), certified nurse midwife (CNM), and certified registered nurse anesthetist (CRNA). The APRN guides the practice and critical thinking of nursing and other healthcare personnel, carries out advanced clinical practice activities, manages one or more clinical practice settings, incorporates scientific knowledge from other disciplines into practice and management, and evaluates the health care provided in those settings through a comprehensive quality assurance system. In the corrections environment, the CNS, NP, or CNM with prescriptive authority often serves as the sole primary care provider. Fewer practice opportunities are currently available for the CRNA. The APRN's practice is characterized by the depth and breadth of knowledge in a nursing specialty and the ability to incorporate knowledge of the correctional field in planning, implementing, and managing health care.

Role Specialty Practice

Corrections nurses may engage in role specialty practice when their primary efforts are focused on education, discharge planning, case management, or administration. Their work most often requires a systems perspective and incorporates fiscal and regulatory considerations in decision-making.

The education and knowledge base acquired at the baccalaureate and master's level prepares corrections nurses to function in administrative roles such as health services managers and chief nurse administrators for large systems. Their clinical expertise, combined with their administrative and managerial training, gives these nurse leaders the depth and breadth of preparation to serve at the senior executive and manager levels to address the inherent political and organizational complexities of the correctional healthcare delivery system.

Educational Preparation and Specialty Certification

Corrections nursing curriculum content and associated clinical practicum experiences are rarely incorporated in formal academic programs at the undergraduate nursing level. If included, most often guest faculty are invited to address care of such vulnerable populations during community health courses. A similar paucity of specific corrections nursing content and specialty practice opportunities characterizes the graduate level educational programs, especially for those preparing registered nurses for the advanced practice roles of clinical nurse specialist, nurse practitioner, and certified nurse midwife. Some academic nursing programs have recently initiated discussions about strategies to formally integrate corrections nursing content or tracks within existing or future curricula.

Nurses interested in the corrections environment may find additional learning opportunities available in college-level criminal justice courses and continuing education and certificate programs offered by such organizations as the American Correctional Association (ACA) and the National Commission on Correctional Health Care (NCCHC). Corrections nurses may also elect to expand their skills and knowledge in other clinical specialty programs of interest such as pediatric, psychiatric–mental health, oncology, hospice and palliative care, or gerontology nursing. Formal preparation for nursing administration roles may be achieved through completion of a graduate-level program in nursing administration. Others may elect to seek advanced degrees in business administration, economics, finance, or law to complement their nursing education preparation and experience.

Certification and advanced certification in correctional health are available through the National Commission on Correctional Health Care. This organization identifies the two types of certification as CCHP for entry level and CCHP-A for the advanced level.

The content in this appendix is not current and is of historical significance only.

In 2006 the American Correctional Association established a certification program for corrections nurses. ACA's Corrections Certification Program is offered in two specialty categories: Certified Corrections Nurse Manager (CCN/M) and Certified Corrections Nurse (CCN).

Certification in nursing administration and other nursing specialties is available through the American Nurses Credentialing Center (ANCC) and other certification bodies. Other certification and credentialing processes may also be recommended or required for specific corrections settings.

Ethics

The registered nurse in the corrections environment is bound by the profession's *Code of Ethics for Nurses with Interpretive Statements* (ANA 2001).

The privacy provision of the Health Insurance Portability and Accountability Act (HIPAA) of 1996 became mandatory in 2003 and has been applied in correctional healthcare systems. Correctional facilities are struggling to determine the relevance and applicability of HIPAA to their operations. Although few state systems have the funds available to support compliance (Orr & Helderstein 2002), the corrections nurse must continue to assure confidentiality and security of patient information, and also advocate for patient privacy as appropriate. Such special regulatory and administrative mandates may create tension as the realities of insufficient fiscal and personnel resources conflict with the rights of the prisoner. For example, medication management and administration may be the responsibility of the guards and other security staff, rather than that of the registered nurse.

By the nature of the practice environment, corrections nurses must consider the primary importance of maintaining public safety. Security issues and concerns are paramount within the correctional institution. Nurses work in partnership with security and correctional staff to assure the provision of appropriate health care to confined individuals. The focus of maintaining security makes correctional nursing practice unique and dynamic, requiring a careful balance of priorities. For example, the person with acute asthma may need immediate access to appropriate inhaler medications to effectively manage their disease. Modifications to the plan of care must be made for the newly diagnosed

The content in this appendix is not current and is of historical significance only.

diabetic patient who needs to learn how to manage their insulin therapy, when needles and syringes cannot be within their assigned berthing area.

The maintenance of professional boundaries is essential in the corrections environment. The nurse must act in the best interest of the patient's medical condition while maintaining a safe and secure environment. Those who cross professional boundaries place themselves, their peers, and others, including the patient, in a position of compromised security and personal safety. These and numerous other issues may merit an ethics consult.

Trends and Issues in Corrections Nursing

Corrections nurses must be advocates for maintaining good conditions of confinement by meeting national standards and monitoring basic needs of daily living in the corrections environment. Constant monitoring of infectious diseases, such as tuberculosis, HIV/AIDS, and hepatitis, in the corrections setting is an important process. Education and prevention become a public health obligation for the corrections nurse in preventing the spread and enhancing the treatment of these infectious diseases in the corrections staff assigned to the facility. This becomes even more important when the incarcerated individual returns to the community and has not yet been cured.

The constitutional right to health care and the changing of community standards of care need to be considered by corrections nurses when developing and reviewing policies in the corrections setting. Research and current practice trends need to be consulted and integrated when appropriate. For example, research supports the use of treatment modalities based on cognitive restructuring to change antisocial behaviors for the corrections populations. These new approaches have significant implications for the corrections nurse working with an aging population, increased numbers of the chronically mentally ill, increased numbers of incarcerated women, and individuals with drug and alcohol abuse.

The increasing numbers of special needs patients, such as those who are chronically ill, elderly, or terminally ill, raise organizational and facility issues that must be addressed. Should elderly and infirm inmates be housed in a separate care setting or be mainstreamed with younger, active, and possibly more aggressive inmates? Prisons are not designed or staffed to provide sophisticated and intensive care for large numbers of chronically ill people. Do new or renovated corrections facilities need to be designed to easily accommodate those with disabilities, such as visual or auditory deficits, or those who are wheelchair-bound or dependent on other mobility assistance?

The managed-care environment is part of corrections nursing. The significant trend of notable budget cuts for health care of inmates is reflective of current times. The frontline corrections nurse manager is charged with maintaining medically necessary care with limited budgetary resources. Nurses are encouraged to uphold the intrinsic values of quality nursing care and to take action if these values are compromised.

The application of telehealth technology has become an enhancement for delivery of healthcare services in the corrections environment. The maintenance of public safety by decreasing movement of patients outside the correctional facility and the practical aspects of making specialist care more readily accessible to more individuals has made the correctional settings a perfect venue for telehealth. This technology solution requires corrections nurses to expand their competencies and knowledge base and also address the resulting documentation and confidentiality issues.

Recruitment and retention of nurses is a challenge for chief nursing officers (CNOs) and administrators in any healthcare setting. This traditional challenge has an even greater impact for the specialty of corrections nursing. Corrections nursing, with its focus on special populations in remote and poorly resourced settings, continues to challenge those desiring to practice in these environments. The pay scale in these settings is often far behind that offered in larger urban settings. Without the recognition and inclusion of corrections nurses in mainstream nursing initiatives, few opportunities exist for nurses to learn about specialization in this area. These challenges can be minimized as corrections nurses align themselves within their specialty and within the larger nursing and healthcare communities. This level of engagement promotes visibility, educates, and bridges the connections between correctional, public, and community health specialties.

Alternative healthcare delivery models include reliance on contracted services of outside agencies rather than department of corrections employees. Because of constraints imposed by mandated bureaucratic county and state hiring practices and set salary scales, these contractors are more successful in recruiting staff to remote areas avoided by nurses and other healthcare professionals. Privatization of inmate healthcare services has the advantage of adjusting salaries to match local wages, providing flexibility to adjust schedules and share staff positions, and hiring temporary staff in times of increased workloads. However, because of the inherent security concerns prevalent in correctional facilities, all nurses require an in-depth orientation to their job assignment, infection control issues, and the security aspects of the institution.

Summary

The corrections nursing specialty allows registered nurses to practice nursing with the compassion and integrity that reflects the essence of nursing. Corrections nurses develop and use strong clinical skills and critical thinking as they manage and respond quickly and decisively when working with this vulnerable population. Nurses utilize their clinical competence, professionalism, and excellent communication skills to deliver high-quality care. Autonomy and independence characterize this practice. The corrections nurse uses negotiation skills that permit positive interactions and effective dialogue with patients and staff in the correctional setting. Such positive interaction allows the nurse to respect the corrections goal of security while promoting patient advocacy and health for this population. Nurses must deliver care in an unbiased and nonjudgmental manner in this challenging environment.

The content in this appendix is not current and is of historical significance only.

STANDARDS OF CORRECTIONS NURSING PRACTICE
STANDARDS OF PRACTICE

The corrections nurse is a registered nurse working in a corrections environment or with confined or detained individuals.

STANDARD 1. ASSESSMENT
The corrections nurse collects comprehensive data pertinent to the patient's health and condition or the situation.

Measurement Criteria:

The corrections nurse:

- Collects data in a systematic and ongoing process.

- Involves the patient, family, and other healthcare and community providers and agencies, as appropriate, in holistic data collection.

- Prioritizes data collection activities based on the patient's immediate condition, the environment of care, and anticipated needs of the patient or situation.

- Uses appropriate evidence-based assessment techniques and instruments in collecting pertinent data.

- Uses analytical models and problem-solving tools.

- Synthesizes available data, information, and knowledge relevant to the situation to identify patterns and variances.

- Documents relevant data in a retrievable format.

Additional Measurement Criteria for the Advanced Practice Registered Nurse:

The advanced practice registered nurse:

- Initiates and interprets diagnostic tests and procedures relevant to the patient's current status.

The content in this appendix is not current and is of historical significance only.

STANDARD 2. DIAGNOSIS
The corrections nurse analyzes the assessment data to determine the diagnoses or issues.

Measurement Criteria:

The corrections nurse:

- Derives the diagnoses or related issues based on assessment data.

- Validates the diagnoses or issues with the patient, family, and other healthcare and community providers when possible and appropriate.

- Documents diagnoses or issues in a manner that facilitates the determination of the expected outcomes and plan.

Additional Measurement Criteria for the Advanced Practice Registered Nurse:

The advanced practice registered nurse:

- Systematically compares clinical findings with normal and abnormal variations and developmental events in formulating a differential diagnosis.

- Utilizes complex data and information obtained during interview, examination, and diagnostic procedures in determining diagnoses.

- Assists staff in developing and maintaining competency in the diagnostic process.

The content in this appendix is not current and is of historical significance only.

STANDARD 3. OUTCOMES IDENTIFICATION
The corrections nurse identifies expected outcomes for a plan individualized to the patient or the situation.

Measurement Criteria:

The corrections nurse:

- Involves the patient, family, and other healthcare and community providers and agencies in formulating expected outcomes when possible and appropriate.

- Derives culturally appropriate expected outcomes from the diagnoses.

- Considers associated risks, security issues, benefits, costs, current scientific evidence, and clinical expertise when formulating expected outcomes.

- Defines expected outcomes in terms of the patient, patient values, ethical considerations, environment, and situation considering associated risks, security issues, benefits and costs, and current scientific evidence.

- Includes a time estimate for attainment of expected outcomes.

- Develops expected outcomes that provide direction for continuity of care.

- Modifies expected outcomes based on changes in the status of the patient or evaluation of the situation.

- Documents expected outcomes as measurable goals.

Additional Measurement Criteria for the Advanced Practice Registered Nurse:

The advanced practice registered nurse:

- Identifies expected outcomes that incorporate cost and clinical effectiveness, patient acceptance, and continuity and consistency among providers.

- Supports the use of clinical guidelines linked to positive patient outcomes.

The content in this appendix is not current and is of historical significance only.

STANDARD 4. PLANNING
The corrections nurse develops a plan that prescribes strategies and alternatives to attain expected outcomes.

Measurement Criteria:

The corrections nurse:

- Develops an individualized plan considering patient characteristics and the situation (e.g., age, gender, cultural appropriateness, environmental sensitivity).

- Develops the plan in conjunction with the patient, family, community and public health resources, security personnel, and others, as appropriate.

- Includes strategies in the plan that address each of the identified diagnoses or issues, which may include strategies for promotion and restoration of health and prevention of illness, injury, and disease.

- Provides for continuity of care within the plan.

- Incorporates an implementation pathway or time line within the plan.

- Establishes the plan priorities with the patient, family, security personnel, and others as appropriate.

- Utilizes the plan to provide direction to other members of the healthcare team and the security personnel.

- Defines the plan to reflect current statutes, rules and regulations, guidelines, and standards.

- Integrates current trends and research affecting care in the planning process.

- Considers the economic impact of the plan.

- Uses standardized language or recognized terminology to document the plan.

The content in this appendix is not current and is of historical significance only.

Additional Measurement Criteria for the Advanced Practice Registered Nurse:

The advanced practice registered nurse:

- Includes assessment, diagnostic strategies, and therapeutic interventions in the plan that reflect current evidence, including data, research, literature, and expert clinical knowledge.

- Selects or designs strategies to meet the multifaceted needs of complex patients.

- Includes the synthesis of the patient's values and beliefs regarding nursing and medical therapies in the plan.

Additional Measurement Criteria for the Nursing Role Specialty:

The corrections nurse in a nursing role specialty:

- Participates in the design and development of multidisciplinary, interdisciplinary, and interagency processes to address the situation or issue.

- Contributes to the development and continuous improvement of organizational systems that support the planning process.

- Supports the integration of clinical, human, financial, and security resources to enhance and complete the decision-making processes.

The content in this appendix is not current and is of historical significance only.

STANDARD 5. IMPLEMENTATION
The corrections nurse implements the identified plan.

Measurement Criteria:

The corrections nurse:

- Implements the plan in a safe and timely manner.
- Documents implementation and any modifications, including changes or omissions, of the identified plan.
- Utilizes evidence-based interventions and treatments specific to the diagnosis or problem.
- Utilizes corrections facility and community resources and systems to implement the plan.
- Collaborates with nursing colleagues, healthcare team members, security personnel, and others to implement the plan.

Additional Measurement Criteria for the Advanced Practice Registered Nurse:

The advanced practice registered nurse:

- Supports collaboration with healthcare colleagues, security personnel, and other disciplines to implement the plan.
- Incorporates new knowledge and strategies to initiate change in healthcare practices if desired outcomes are not achieved.

Additional Measurement Criteria for the Nursing Role Specialty:

The corrections nurse in a nursing role specialty:

- Facilitates utilization of systems and community resources to implement the plan.
- Implements the plan using principles and concepts of project or systems management.
- Fosters organizational systems that support implementation of the plan.

STANDARD 5A. COORDINATION OF CARE
The corrections nurse coordinates care delivery.

Measurement Criteria:

The corrections nurse:

- Coordinates implementation of the plan.
- Employs strategies to promote health and a safe and secure environment.
- Documents the coordination of care.

Measurement Criteria for the Advanced Practice Registered Nurse:

The advanced practice registered nurse:

- Provides leadership in the coordination of multidisciplinary health care for integrated delivery of patient care services.
- Synthesizes data and information in order to prescribe necessary system and community support measures, including environmental modifications.
- Coordinates system and community resources that enhance delivery of care across continuums.

Measurement Criteria for the Nurse in the Role Specialty:

The corrections nurse in a nursing role specialty:

- Coordinates system and community resources that enhance delivery of care across continuums.
- Evaluates fiscal impact and needs when making decisions related to the delivery of care.

The content in this appendix is not current and is of historical significance only.

STANDARD 5B. HEALTH TEACHING AND HEALTH PROMOTION
The corrections nurse employs strategies to promote health and a safe environment.

Measurement Criteria:

The corrections nurse:

- Provides health teaching to patients, family, colleagues, and security personnel that addresses such topics as healthy lifestyles, risk-reducing behaviors, developmental needs, activities of daily living, and preventive self-care.

- Uses health promotion and health teaching methods appropriate to the situation and the patient's developmental level, learning needs, readiness, ability to learn, language preference, and culture.

- Seeks opportunities for feedback and evaluation of the effectiveness of the strategies used.

Additional Measurement Criteria for the Advanced Practice Registered Nurse:

The advanced practice registered nurse:

- Synthesizes empirical evidence on risk behaviors, epidemiology, and other related theories and frameworks when designing health information and patient education.

- Designs patient education appropriate to the patient's developmental level, learning needs, readiness to learn, and cultural values and beliefs.

Additional Measurement Criteria for the Nursing Role Specialty:

The corrections nurse in a nursing role specialty:

- Synthesizes empirical evidence on risk behaviors, learning theories, behavioral change theories, motivational theories, epidemiology, and other related theories and frameworks when designing health information and patient education.

- Designs health information and patient education appropriate to the patient's developmental level, learning needs, readiness to learn, and cultural values and beliefs.

The content in this appendix is not current and is of historical significance only.

- Designs, implements, and supports health teaching that addresses chronic illness, communicable disease, access to health care, and emergency care specific for the corrections environment.

- Evaluates health information resources, such as the Internet, within the area of practice for accuracy, readability, and comprehensibility to help patients access quality health information.

The content in this appendix is not current and is of historical significance only.

Standard 5c. Consultation

The advanced practice registered nurse and the nursing role specialist provide consultation to influence the identified plan, enhance the abilities of others, and effect change.

Measurement Criteria for the Advanced Practice Registered Nurse:

The advanced practice registered nurse:

- Synthesizes clinical data, theoretical frameworks, and evidence when providing consultation.

- Facilitates the effectiveness of a consultation by involving the patient in decision-making and negotiating role responsibilities.

- Communicates consultation recommendations that facilitate change.

Measurement Criteria for the Nursing Role Specialty:

The corrections nurse in a nursing role specialty:

- Synthesizes data, information, theoretical frameworks, and evidence when providing consultation.

- Facilitates the effectiveness of a consultation by involving the stakeholders in the decision-making process.

- Communicates consultation recommendations that influence the identified plan, facilitate understanding by involved stakeholders, enhance the work of others, and effect change.

The content in this appendix is not current and is of historical significance only.

STANDARD 5D. PRESCRIPTIVE AUTHORITY AND TREATMENT
The advanced practice registered nurse uses prescriptive authority, procedures, referrals, treatments, and therapies in accordance with state and federal laws and regulations.

Measurement Criteria for the Advanced Practice Registered Nurse:

The advanced practice registered nurse:

- Prescribes evidence-based treatments, therapies, and procedures considering the patient's comprehensive healthcare needs.

- Prescribes pharmacological agents based on a current knowledge of pharmacology and physiology.

- Prescribes specific pharmacological agents and treatments based on clinical indicators, the patient's status and needs, and the results of diagnostic and laboratory tests.

- Evaluates therapeutic and potential adverse effects of pharmacological and non-pharmacological treatments.

- Provides patients with information about intended effects and potential adverse effects of proposed prescriptive therapies.

- Provides information about costs and alternative treatments and procedures, as appropriate.

The content in this appendix is not current and is of historical significance only.

STANDARD 6. EVALUATION

The corrections nurse evaluates progress towards attainment of outcomes.

Measurement Criteria:

The corrections nurse:

- Conducts a systematic, ongoing, and criterion-based evaluation of the outcomes in relation to the structures and processes prescribed by the plan and the indicated time line.

- Includes the patient and others involved in the care or situation in the evaluative process.

- Evaluates the effectiveness of the planned strategies in relation to patient responses and the attainment of the expected outcomes.

- Documents the results of the evaluation.

- Uses ongoing assessment data to revise the diagnoses, outcomes, plan, and implementation as needed.

- Disseminates the results to the patient and others involved in the care or situation, as appropriate, in accordance with state and federal laws and regulations.

Additional Measurement Criteria for the Advanced Practice Registered Nurse:

The advanced practice registered nurse:

- Evaluates the accuracy of the diagnosis and effectiveness of the interventions in relation to the patient's attainment of expected outcomes.

- Synthesizes the results of the evaluation analyses to determine the impact of the plan on the affected patients, families, groups, communities, and corrections and other institutions.

- Uses the results of the evaluation analyses to make or recommend process or structural changes including policy, procedure, or protocol documentation, as appropriate.

The content in this appendix is not current and is of historical significance only.

Additional Measurement Criteria for the Nursing Role Specialty:

The corrections nurse in a nursing role specialty:

- Uses the results of the evaluation analyses to make or recommend process or structural changes, including policy, procedure, regulation, and legislation, or protocol documentation, as appropriate.

- Synthesizes the results of the evaluation analyses to determine the impact of the plan on the affected patients, families, groups, communities, and corrections and other institutions, networks, and organizations.

This page left intentionally blank.

The content in this appendix is not current and is of historical significance only.

STANDARDS OF PROFESSIONAL PERFORMANCE

The corrections nurse is a registered nurse working in a corrections environment or with confined or detained individuals.

STANDARD 7. QUALITY OF PRACTICE
The corrections nurse systematically enhances the quality and effectiveness of nursing practice.

Measurement Criteria:

The corrections nurse:

- Demonstrates quality by documenting the application of the nursing process in a responsible, accountable, and ethical manner.

- Uses creativity and innovation in nursing practice to improve care delivery.

- Incorporates new knowledge to initiate changes in nursing practice if desired outcomes are not achieved.

- Participates in quality improvement activities. Such activities may include:

  - Identifying aspects of practice important for quality monitoring.

  - Using indicators developed to monitor quality and effectiveness of nursing practice.

  - Collecting data to monitor quality and effectiveness of nursing practice.

  - Analyzing quality data to identify opportunities for improving nursing practice.

  - Formulating recommendations to improve nursing practice or outcomes.

  - Implementing activities to enhance the quality of nursing practice.

  - Developing, implementing, and evaluating policies, procedures, and guidelines to improve the quality of practice.

Continued ▶

The content in this appendix is not current and is of historical significance only.

- Participating on interdisciplinary teams to evaluate clinical care or health services.

- Participating in efforts to minimize costs and unnecessary duplication.

- Analyzing factors related to safety, satisfaction, effectiveness, and cost–benefit options.

- Analyzing organizational systems for barriers.

- Implementing processes that promote optimal, safe, and effective care.

- Uses the results of quality improvement activities to initiate changes in nursing practice, healthcare delivery, and the correctional system.

Additional Measurement Criteria for the Advanced Practice Registered Nurse:

The advanced practice registered nurse:

- Obtains and maintains professional certification if available in the area of expertise.

- Designs quality improvement initiatives.

- Implements initiatives to evaluate the need for change.

- Evaluates the practice environment and quality of nursing care rendered in relation to existing evidence, identifying opportunities for the generation and use of research.

Additional Measurement Criteria for the Nursing Role Specialty:

The corrections nurse in a nursing role specialty:

- Obtains and maintains professional certification if available in the area of expertise.

- Designs quality improvement initiatives.

- Implements initiatives to evaluate the need for change.

- Evaluates the practice environment, including the quality of nursing care, in relation to existing evidence, identifying opportunities for improvement, including the generation and use of research.

STANDARD 8. EDUCATION
The corrections nurse attains knowledge and competency that reflects current nursing practice.

Measurement Criteria:

The corrections nurse:

- Participates in ongoing educational activities related to appropriate knowledge bases and professional issues.

- Demonstrates a commitment to lifelong learning through self-reflection and inquiry to identify learning needs.

- Seeks experiences that reflect current practice in order to maintain skills and competence in clinical practice or role performance.

- Acquires knowledge and skills appropriate to the specialty area, practice setting, role, or situation.

- Maintains professional records that provide evidence of competency and lifelong learning.

- Seeks experiences and formal and independent learning activities to maintain and develop clinical and professional skills and knowledge.

Additional Measurement Criteria for the Advanced Practice Registered Nurse:

The advanced practice registered nurse:

- Uses current healthcare research findings and other evidence to expand clinical knowledge, enhance role performance, and increase knowledge of professional issues.

Additional Measurement Criteria for the Nursing Role Specialty:

The corrections nurse in a nursing role specialty:

- Uses current research findings and other evidence to expand knowledge, enhance role performance, and increase knowledge of professional and leadership issues.

The content in this appendix is not current and is of historical significance only.

STANDARD 9. PROFESSIONAL PRACTICE EVALUATION
The corrections nurse evaluates one's own nursing practice in relation to professional practice standards and guidelines, relevant statutes, rules, and regulations.

Measurement Criteria:

The corrections nurse's practice reflects the application of knowledge of current practice standards, guidelines, statutes, rules, and regulations.

The corrections nurse:

- Provides nursing care considering age, culture, ethnicity, and the unique aspects of the correctional environment.

- Engages in self-evaluation of practice on a regular basis, identifying areas of strength as well as areas in which professional development would be beneficial.

- Obtains informal feedback regarding one's own practice from patients, peers, professional colleagues, and others.

- Participates in systematic peer review as appropriate.

- Takes action to achieve goals identified during the evaluation process.

- Provides rationales for practice beliefs, decisions, and actions as part of the informal and formal evaluation processes.

Additional Measurement Criteria for the Advanced Practice Registered Nurse:

The advanced practice registered nurse:

- Engages in a formal process seeking feedback regarding one's own practice from patients, peers, professional colleagues, and others.

Additional Measurement Criteria for the Nursing Role Specialty:

The corrections nurse in a nursing role specialty:

- Engages in a formal process seeking feedback regarding role performance from individuals; professional colleagues; representatives and administrators of corrections, government, or corporate entities; and others.

The content in this appendix is not current and is of historical significance only.

STANDARD 10. COLLEGIALITY
The corrections nurse interacts with and contributes to the professional development of peers and colleagues.

Measurement Criteria:

The corrections nurse:

- Shares knowledge and skills with peers and colleagues as evidenced by such activities as patient care conferences or presentations at formal or informal meetings.
- Provides peers with feedback regarding their practice and role performance.
- Interacts with peers and colleagues to enhance one's own professional nursing practice and role performance.
- Maintains compassionate and caring relationships with peers and colleagues.
- Contributes to an environment that is conducive to the education of healthcare professionals.
- Contributes to a supportive and healthy work environment.

Additional Measurement Criteria for the Advanced Practice Registered Nurse:

The advanced practice registered nurse:

- Models expert practice to interdisciplinary team members and healthcare consumers.
- Mentors and precepts other corrections nurses and colleagues as appropriate.
- Participates with interdisciplinary teams that contribute to role development and advanced nursing practice and health care.

Additional Measurement Criteria for the Nursing Role Specialty:

The corrections nurse in a nursing role specialty:

- Participates on multidisciplinary teams that contribute to role development and, directly or indirectly, advance nursing practice and health services.
- Mentors and precepts other corrections nurses and colleagues, as appropriate.

The content in this appendix is not current and is of historical significance only.

STANDARD 11. COLLABORATION
The corrections nurse collaborates with patient, family, and others in the conduct of nursing practice.

Measurement Criteria:

The corrections nurse:

- Communicates with patient, family, healthcare providers, and corrections staff regarding patient care and the nurse's role in the provision of that care.

- Collaborates in creating a documented plan focused on outcomes and decisions related to care and delivery of services that indicates communication with patients, families, and others.

- Partners with others to effect change and generate positive outcomes through knowledge of the patient or situation.

- Documents referrals, including provisions for continuity of care.

Additional Measurement Criteria for the Advanced Practice Registered Nurse:

The advanced practice registered nurse:

- Partners with other disciplines to enhance patient care through interdisciplinary activities such as education, consultation, management, technological development, and research opportunities.

- Facilitates an interdisciplinary process with other members of the healthcare team.

- Documents plan of care communications, rationales for plan of care changes, and collaborative discussions to improve patient care.

Additional Measurement Criteria for Nursing Role Specialty:

The corrections nurse in a nursing role specialty:

- Works with others to enhance health care, and ultimately patient care, through interdisciplinary activities such as education, consultation, management, technological development, and research opportunities.

The content in this appendix is not current and is of historical significance only.

- Facilitates an interdisciplinary process with corrections staff and community resources.
- Documents plans, communications, rationales for plan changes, and collaborative discussions.

The content in this appendix is not current and is of historical significance only.

STANDARD 12. ETHICS

The corrections nurse integrates ethical provisions in all areas of practice.

Measurement Criteria:

The corrections nurse:

- Uses *Code of Ethics for Nurses with Interpretive Statements* (ANA 2001) to guide practice.

- Delivers care in a manner that preserves and protects patient autonomy, dignity, and rights.

- Maintains patient confidentiality within legal and regulatory parameters considering the unique corrections environment.

- Serves as a patient advocate and assists patients in developing skills for self-advocacy.

- Maintains a therapeutic and professional patient–nurse relationship with appropriate professional role boundaries.

- Demonstrates a commitment to practicing self-care, managing stress, and connecting with self and others.

- Contributes to resolving ethical issues of patients, colleagues, or systems as evidenced in such activities as participating on ethics committees.

- Reports illegal, incompetent, or impaired practices.

Additional Measurement Criteria for the Advanced Practice Registered Nurse:

The advanced practice registered nurse:

- Informs the patient of the risks, benefits, and outcomes of health-care regimens.

- Participates in interdisciplinary teams that address ethical risks, benefits, and outcomes.

The content in this appendix is not current and is of historical significance only.

Additional Measurement Criteria for the Nursing Role Specialty:

The corrections nurse in a nursing role specialty:

- Participates in multidisciplinary and interdisciplinary teams that address ethical risks, benefits, and outcomes.

- Informs administrators or others of the risks, benefits, and outcomes of programs and decisions that affect healthcare delivery.

The content in this appendix is not current and is of historical significance only.

STANDARD 13. RESEARCH
The corrections nurse integrates research findings into practice.

Measurement Criteria:

The corrections nurse:

- Utilizes the best available evidence, including research findings, to guide practice decisions.

- Actively participates in research activities at various levels appropriate to the nurse's level of education and position. Such activities may include:

  - Identifying clinical problems specific to nursing research (patient care and nursing practice);

  - Participating in data collection (surveys, pilot projects, formal studies);

  - Participating in a formal committee or program;

  - Sharing research activities or findings with peers and others;

  - Conducting research;

  - Critically analyzing and interpreting research for application to practice;

  - Using research findings in the development of policies, procedures, and standards of practice in patient care; and

  - Incorporating research as a basis for learning.

- Recognizes the unique requirements of human subjects' protection in the corrections environment.

Additional Measurement Criteria for the Advanced Practice Registered Nurse:

The advanced practice registered nurse:

- Contributes to nursing knowledge by conducting or synthesizing research that discovers, examines, and evaluates knowledge, theories, criteria, and creative approaches to improve healthcare practice, especially in the corrections environment.

- Formally disseminates research findings through activities such as presentations, publications, consultation, and journal clubs.

The content in this appendix is not current and is of historical significance only.

Additional Measurement Criteria for the Nursing Role Specialty:

The corrections nurse in a nursing role specialty:

- Contributes to nursing knowledge by conducting or synthesizing research that discovers, examines, and evaluates knowledge, theories, criteria, and creative approaches to improve health care.

- Formally disseminates research findings through activities such as presentations, publications, consultation, and journal clubs.

The content in this appendix is not current and is of historical significance only.

STANDARD 14. RESOURCE UTILIZATION

The corrections nurse considers factors related to safety, effectiveness, cost, benefits, and impact on practice in the planning and delivery of nursing services.

Measurement Criteria:

The corrections nurse:

- Evaluates factors such as safety, security, effectiveness, availability, cost and benefits, efficiencies, and impact on practice when choosing practice options that would result in the same expected outcome.

- Assists the patient, family, corrections staff, and community resource personnel in identifying and securing appropriate and available services to address health-related needs.

- Assigns or delegates tasks, based on the needs and condition of the patient, potential for harm, stability of the patient's condition, complexity of the task, and predictability of the outcome.

- Assists the patient and family in becoming informed consumers about the options, risks, and benefits of treatment and care.

Additional Measurement Criteria for the Advanced Practice Registered Nurse:

The advanced practice registered nurse:

- Utilizes organizational and community resources to formulate multidisciplinary or interdisciplinary plans of care.

- Develops innovative solutions for patient care problems that address effective resource utilization and maintenance of quality.

- Develops evaluation strategies to demonstrate cost-effectiveness, cost–benefit, and efficiency factors associated with clinical practice.

Additional Measurement Criteria for the Nursing Role Specialty:

The corrections nurse in a nursing role specialty:

- Develops innovative solutions and applies strategies to obtain appropriate resources for nursing initiatives.

- Secures organizational resources to ensure a work environment conducive to completing the identified plan and outcomes.

The content in this appendix is not current and is of historical significance only.

- Develops evaluation methods to measure safety, security, and effectiveness for interventions and outcomes.

- Promotes activities that assist others, as appropriate, in becoming informed about costs, risks, and benefits of care or of the plan and treatment strategies.

The content in this appendix is not current and is of historical significance only.

Standard 15. Leadership

The corrections nurse provides leadership in the professional practice setting and the profession.

Measurement Criteria:

The corrections nurse:

- Engages in teamwork as a team player and a team builder.

- Works to create and maintain healthy work environments in local, regional, national, or international communities.

- Displays the ability to define a clear vision, associated goals, and a plan to implement and measure progress.

- Demonstrates a commitment to continuous, lifelong learning for self and others.

- Teaches others to succeed, by mentoring and other strategies.

- Exhibits creativity and flexibility through times of change.

- Demonstrates energy, excitement, and a passion for quality work.

- Willingly accepts mistakes by self and others, thereby creating a culture in which risk-taking is not only safe, but expected.

- Inspires loyalty through valuing of people as the most precious assets in an organization.

- Directs the coordination of care across settings and among caregivers, including oversight of licensed and unlicensed personnel in any assigned or delegated tasks.

- Serves in key roles in the work setting by participating in committees, councils, and administrative teams.

- Promotes advancement of the profession through participation in professional organizations.

Additional Measurement Criteria for the Advanced Practice Registered Nurse:

The advanced practice registered nurse:

- Works to influence decision-making bodies to improve patient care.

- Provides direction to enhance the effectiveness of the healthcare team.

- Initiates and revises protocols or guidelines to reflect evidence-based practice, to reflect accepted changes in care management, or to address emerging problems.

- Promotes communication of information and advancement of the profession through writing, publishing, and presentations for professional or lay audiences.

- Designs innovations to effect change in practice and improve health outcomes.

Additional Measurement Criteria for the Nursing Role Specialty:

The corrections nurse in a nursing role specialty:

- Works to influence decision-making bodies to improve patient care, health services, delivery systems, and organizational and governmental policies.

- Promotes communication of information and advancement of the profession through writing, publishing, and presentations for professional or lay audiences.

- Designs innovations to effect change in practice and outcomes.

- Provides direction to enhance the effectiveness of the multi-disciplinary or interdisciplinary team.

The content in this appendix is not current and is of historical significance only.

GLOSSARY

Assessment. A systematic, dynamic process by which the corrections nurse through interaction with the patient, family, groups, communities, public health agencies, populations, and healthcare providers, collects and analyzes data. Assessment may include the following dimensions: physical, psychological, sociocultural, spiritual, cognitive, functional abilities, developmental, economic, and lifestyle.

Caregiver. A person who provides direct care for another, such as a child, a dependent adult, or a person who is disabled or chronically ill.

Code of ethics. A list of provisions that makes explicit the primary goals, values, and obligations of the profession.

Community. Local health jurisdictions, health departments, hospitals, and similar entities; urgent care and emergency departments.

Continuity of care. An interdisciplinary process that includes patients, families, and significant others in the development of a coordinated plan of care. This process facilitates the patient's transition between settings and healthcare providers, based on changing needs and available resources.

Corrections environment. A facility or place of confinement that houses offender, detainee, or convicted clientele.

Corrections nurse. A registered nurse who works in a corrections environment or with confined or detained individuals.

Corrections nursing. The practice of nursing and the delivery of care within the unique and distinct environment of the criminal justice system. The criminal justice system includes jails, prisons, juvenile detention centers, substance abuse treatment facilities, and other facilities.

Criteria. Relevant, measurable indicators of the standards of practice and professional performance.

Data. Discrete entities that are described objectively without interpretation.

Diagnosis. A clinical judgment about the patient's response to actual or potential health conditions or needs. The diagnosis provides the basis

The content in this appendix is not current and is of historical significance only.

for determination of a plan to achieve expected outcomes. Corrections nurses utilize nursing and/or medical diagnoses, depending upon educational and clinical preparation and legal authority.

Disease. A biological or psychosocial disorder of structure or function in a patient, especially one that produces specific signs or symptoms or that affects a specific part of the body, mind, or spirit.

Environment. The atmosphere, milieu, or conditions in which an individual lives, works, or plays.

Evaluation. The process of determining the progress toward attainment of expected outcomes, including the effectiveness of care, when addressing one's practice.

Evidence-based practice. A process founded on the collection, interpretation, and integration of valid, important, and applicable patient-reported, clinician-observed, and research-derived evidence. The best available evidence, moderated by patient circumstances and preferences, is applied to improve the quality of clinical judgments.

Expected outcomes. End results that are measurable, desirable, observable, and which translate into observable behaviors.

Family. Family of origin or significant others as identified by the patient.

Guidelines. Systematically developed statements that describe recommended actions based on available scientific evidence and expert opinion. Clinical guidelines describe a process of patient care management that has the potential of improving the quality of clinical and consumer decision-making.

Health. An experience that is often expressed in terms of wellness and illness and which may occur in the presence or absence of disease or injury.

Healthcare providers. Individuals with special expertise who provide healthcare services or assistance to patients. They may include nurses, physicians, psychologists, social workers, nutritionists/dietitians, and various therapists.

Holistic. An understanding that the parts of a patient are intimately interconnected and that physical, mental, social, and spiritual factors need to be included in any interventions.

The content in this appendix is not current and is of historical significance only.

Illness. The subjective experience of discomfort.

Implementation. Activities such as teaching, monitoring, providing, counseling, delegating, and coordinating.

Information. Data that are interpreted, organized, or structured.

Interdisciplinary. Using the overlapping skills and knowledge of each team member and discipline resulting in synergistic effects where outcomes are enhanced and are more comprehensive than the simple aggregation of any team member's individual efforts.

Knowledge. Information that is synthesized so that relationships are identified and formalized.

Multidisciplinary. Using the contribution of discipline-specific skills by each team member or discipline.

Patient. Recipient of nursing practice. The term *patient* is used to provide consistency and brevity, bearing in mind that other terms such as client, individual, resident, family, groups, communities, or populations might be better choices in some instances. When the patient is an individual, the focus is on the health state, problems, or needs of the individual. When the patient is a family or group, the focus is on the health state of the unit as a whole or the reciprocal effects of the individual's health state on the other members of the unit. When the patient is a community or population, the focus is on personal and environmental health and the health risks of the community or population.

Peer review. A collegial, systematic, and periodic process by which health professionals are held accountable for practice and which fosters the refinement of one's knowledge, skills, and decision-making at all levels and in all areas of practice.

Plan. A comprehensive outline of the components that need to be addressed to attain expected outcomes.

Quality of care. The degree to which health services for patients, families, groups, communities, or populations increase the likelihood of desired outcomes and are consistent with current professional knowledge.

Situation. A set of circumstances, conditions, or events.

Stakeholders. Persons who are affected by and care about the outcome or situation; may include patients, families, communities, corrections staff, healthcare providers, and others.

The content in this appendix is not current and is of historical significance only.

Standard. An authoritative statement defined and promoted by the profession, by which the quality of practice, service, or education can be evaluated.

Strategy. A plan of action to achieve a major overall goal.

Time line. A chronology for the plan of action to achieve a major overall goal.

The content in this appendix is not current and is of historical significance only.

REFERENCES

American Correctional Association (ACA). 2004. Female offenders. [survey]. *Corrections Compendium 29*:(3). (May/June). White Plains, MD: ACA.

American Correctional Association. 2005a. *2005 Directory of adult and juvenile correctional departments, institutions, agencies, probation and parole authorities.* White Plains, MD: ACA.

American Correctional Association. 2005b. *Corrections Compendium 29*:(5). (September/October). White Plains, MD: ACA.

American Nurses Association (ANA). 2001. *Code of ethics for nurses with interpretive statements.* Washington, DC: American Nurses Publishing.

American Nurses Association (ANA). 2003. *Nursing's social policy statement, 2nd ed.* Washington, DC: Nursesbooks.org.

American Nurses Association (ANA). 2004. *Nursing: Scope and standards of practice.* Silver Spring, MD: Nursesbooks.org.

American Public Health Association (APHA). 2003. *Standards for health services in correctional institutions.* Washington, DC: APHA.

Anno, B. J. 1997. Health behaviors in prisons and correctional facilities, in *Handbook of health behaviors research, Vol. III: Demography, development, and diversity,* Ch. 14, ed. David S. Gochman. New York: Plenum Press.

Anno, B. J., C. Graham, J. E. Lawrence, & R. Shansky. 2004. *Correctional health care: Addressing the needs of elderly, chronically Ill, and terminally ill inmates.* Washington, DC: Criminal Justice Institute, National Institute of Corrections. http://www.nicic.org/Downloads/PDF/2004/018735.pdf (accessed January 4, 2007).

Bureau of Justice Statistics. 2004. *Corrections statistics.* Washington, DC: Department of Justice. http://www.ojp.usdoj.gov/bjs/correct.htm (accessed January 4, 2007).

The content in this appendix is not current and is of historical significance only.

Estelle v. Gamble, 429 U.S. 97. 1976. Washington, DC: U.S. Supreme Court (available online). http://www.caselaw.lp.findlaw.com

Goldkuhle, U. 1999. Health service utilization by women in prison: Health needs indicators and response effects. *Journal of Correctional Health Care* 1:63–83.

Greenfeld, L. A., & T. L. Snell. 1999. *Women offenders*. Washington, DC: U.S. Department of Justice, Bureau of Justice Statistics.

MacNeil, J. 2005. An unanswered health disparity: TB among correctional inmates: 1993–2003. *American Journal of Public Health* cited on www.medicalnewstoday.com/medicalnews.php?.newsid=31801 (accessed January 4, 2007).

Murtha, R. 1975. Changes in one city's system. *American Journal of Nursing 75*(3):421–22.

National Commission on Correctional Health Care (NCCHC). 2002. *The health status of soon-to-be-released inmates*. Washington, DC: NCCHC. http://www.ncchc.org/pubs/pubs_stbr.vol1.html (accessed January 4, 2007).

Orr, D., & D. Helderstein. 2002. HIPAA in state correctional systems. *Journal of Correctional Health Care 9*(3):345–59.

National Criminal Justice Reference Service. 2003. *Sourcebook of criminal justice statistics online, 31st ed*. Albany, NY: U.S. Department of Justice, Bureau of Justice Statistics, Hindelang Criminal Justice Research Center. http://www.albany.edu/sourcebook/ (accessed January 4, 2007).

U.S. Department of Health and Human Services (USDHHS). 2002. *The registered nurse population: Findings from the national sample survey of registered nurses, March 2000*. Washington, DC: USDHHS, Health Resource and Services Administration, Bureau of Health Professions, Division of Nursing. http://bhpr.hrsa.gov/healthworkforce/reports/rnsurvey/default.htm (accessed January 6, 2007).

U.S. Department of Justice (USDOJ). 2004. *Juvenile offenders and victims national report series*. http://www.ncjrs.gov/pdffiles1/ojjdp/202885.pdf (accessed January 4, 2007).

Index

Note: Entries with [2007] indicate an entry from *Corrections Nursing: Scope and Standards of Practice* (2007), reproduced in Appendix A. That information is not current but included for historical value only.

A

Abilities in correctional nursing practice, 1, 9, 14–15, 16, 22, 31, 44, 46, 52, 53, 59, 84, 87, 90, 103, 105, 123
See also Knowledge, skills, abilities, and judgment

ACA. *See* American Corrections Association (ACA)

Academy of Correctional Health Professionals, 25, 84

Accessibility to health care and nursing practice, 3, 4, 5, 9, 10, 11, 12, 21, 22, 41, 44, 45, 77, 78`, 84, 104

Accountability in correctional nursing practice, 3, 12–13, 19, 22, 77
leadership and, 58
quality of practice and, 55
safety and security and, 12–13
See also Delegation; Responsibility

ACHSA. *See* American Correctional Health Services Association (ACHSA)

Activities in correctional nursing practice
educational, 52
health promotion, 11, 45

interprofessional, 61
security, 12–13

Acute care in correctional settings, 10–11

Administration in correctional nursing practice, 12, 13, 17, 23
certification, 25
education, 24
ethics, 20
technology and, 28

Administrative segregation, 29–30

Adult population, 5, 6, 7, 10, 27, 28, 80, 81
See also Older inmates

Advanced practice registered nurses (APRNs) in correctional nursing practice, 4, 9, 10, 22–23
assessment competencies, 35
measurement criteria [2007], 96
collaboration competencies, 61
measurement criteria [2007], 115
collegiality competencies
measurement criteria [2007], 114
consultation competencies, 46
measurement criteria [2007], 105